Changing Focus

Changing Focus

*From Left Brain Thinking
to Right Brain "Being"*

Patricia Fraser

HybridGlobal
PUBLISHING

Published by
Hybrid Global Publishing
301 E 57th Street, 4th fl
New York, NY 10022

Manufactured in the United States of America, or in the
United Kingdom when distributed elsewhere.

Fraser, Patricia
Changing Focus: From Left Brain Thinking to Right Brain "Being"
LCCN: 2019934302
ISBN: 9781948181471
eBook: 9781948181488

Cover design by: Joe Potter
Copyediting: Linda Atherton
Interior design: Medlar Publishing Solutions Pvt Ltd., India

Dedication

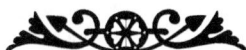

dedicate this book to the late Professor James H. Hargreaves. Jim, you greatly influenced my creative and intellectual development. I think of you often. Also, I dedicate this book to the late Mary Duggan Barkhouse. Mary, your generous and loving spirit inspired me to become a writer. Your spirit is still with me. Finally, I dedicate this book to Abby, Kia, Leila, and Maison. You guys are the best. Thank you so much for being so honest and sweet.

Contents

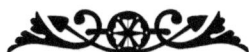

	Introduction	ix
CHAPTER 1	Love Is Our Purpose	1
CHAPTER 2	Right Brain/Left Brain	13
CHAPTER 3	Creativity	29
CHAPTER 4	L-Mode Thinking	45
CHAPTER 5	The Subtle Reality of Existence	65
CHAPTER 6	Negative Influences	83
CHAPTER 7	Loneliness and Being Alone	99
CHAPTER 8	Our True Selves	113
CHAPTER 9	Letting Go	127
CHAPTER 10	Changing Focus	139

Introduction

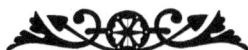

Life is a creative process. I've always understood this on some level, but learning to clarify and verbalize this idea has taken me many years. "Changing Focus" is the result of my continuous search for answers about the connection between creativity and spirituality.

I have been studying music and art since I was a child and have a degree in both Music and Education. As an artist and educator, I have been fascinated by the incredibly positive effects of studying "the arts". This fascination grew when, in the early 80's, I read a book titled "Drawing on the Right Side of the Brain" by a woman named Betty Edwards. This book caused me to change the way I view life and "the arts" and is what prompted me to search for a way to express the connection between the creative process and spiritual evolution.

"Drawing on the Right Side of the Brain" explains some of the differences between the way the right and left hemispheres of the brain process information or perceive reality. Dr. Edwards' book teaches the reader how to improve their ability to draw realistic art by instructing them on how to use the right brain. When I studied the book, I was struck by the fact that it caused immediate improvement in my drawing ability and was fascinated by the information it gave about the creative process. This information caused me to feel certain that there is a connection between the spirit and the creative right brain, and I have since then developed and refined this idea. The secret in drawing, but also in spiritual evolution, is to become aware of the two brain modes and learn to shift from one to the other.

"Changing Focus" explores and exposes the left/right shift in the context of love, creativity and art, thinking, our daily physical existence, and of course our spiritual evolution. The purpose of the book is to help us understand more about the role our creative right brain plays in our spiritual evolution. Once we learn how to change focus from the dominant, controlling logic of left mode thinking, to the creative ways of the right brain, we can use these new skills to become more aware of the subtle reality of spirit.

CHAPTER 1

Love Is Our Purpose

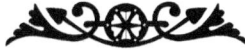

I f we believe we are spiritual beings in a physical existence, why don't we remember this or feel a connection to spirit at all times? The biggest reason why we lose our connection to spirit is because we spend most of our time in a left brain, logic based state. When we have to have logical proof for everything, how can we believe something as abstract as a spiritual essence, or God, or a universal plan? How can we possibly remember our essence? We remember it by learning to appreciate, absorb, flow with, and trust the subtle part of reality through the use of our creative mind. When we shift our way of viewing life from a logic base to a creative base, we begin to see the subtle aspect of reality that underlies everything.

My childhood was filled with opportunities to develop my creative mind. I have always loved to draw. As a child I would spend hours on a single drawing trying to make sure I had included every small detail I could see. I loved these drawing experiences because they were so relaxing and interesting. Also, I come from a family that greatly respects music. In the late 50's, when television was becoming popular, my parents held back on purchasing one because they wanted to spend any extra money they had on something that they considered to be a priority. Instead of a television they bought a piano and made sure that my siblings and I took piano lessons as soon as we were old enough to do so. My mother also taught us to sing as a group. We performed at concerts and other events in our community and spent many hours practicing at home. I grew up treating music with respect. It became a very important part of my life. Through the music department at our local university, I was able to receive classical training in flute and to broaden my exposure to creative people and situations.

All of these experiences helped me to expand the use of my creative mind. I was training myself to really listen and to really see. I was learning how to notice the subtle changes and patterns of sounds and visual images. This training was enhanced by experiences I had with nature. One of the greatest things about growing up where I did was the fact that we were very close to the ocean. We lived at our cottage during the summers, and that gave me the opportunity to make a strong connection with nature. I learned how to become absorbed in the beauty around me and how to feel comfortable being alone. When I was sitting alone watching the waves, smelling the salt air, or listening to the sounds that surrounded me, I was learning to let my creative mind carry me into the subtle beauty of nature. I was uniting with nature by appreciating its beauty.

Creativity and nature can sharpen our senses so that we hear, smell, feel, see and taste subtle beauty. When we unite emotionally with this subtle beauty, we are uniting with universal love. Emotional unity with universal love gives us truths and insights that remove us from a logic based view of life.

All of life is governed, guided, and enlightened by a unified force. All that exists is made from this energy of life. The way we experience this unified field is by connecting to it in the form of love. Universal love, our essential nature, is what we are here to discover. We have to define love in its gross forms and increase our understanding of it in its most subtle forms. This is our purpose. Once we understand the real nature of love, we discover that it gives us our power. When we are filled with the emotions and awareness of love, our heart opens, our mind clears, our fears lessen, and we feel heard, understood, supported, guided, and utterly thankful for and in love with life.

Getting to know love is a complex process, especially if you do not have a clear understanding of the different modes our brain has of perceiving reality. So, in our search for understanding of and connection to love, we have to include a study of how we've been trained to use our brain. Love is our purpose. The creative mind aids the process of discovering the subtle essence of love.

Normally, we define love based on our experiences of loving others and being loved. I suppose the most complete love many of us have experienced is the overwhelming emotions of love you feel for your newborn child. For a day or so after my daughter was born, I felt as though her and I were the only people in my life. I was so struck with feelings of love and awe that all I could do was think of her. Sometimes it takes a while for this type of bond to be formed, and other times it happens as soon as your child is born. Either way, a parental bond can be extremely intense. I'm sure this love occurs because babies are so helpless and innocent. They receive our love because it pours out of us. We don't choose to love them. We react instinctively, and this love feels very pure. This is probably the most instinctive love response most of us have experienced.

While this love is completely pure, we know from experience that love can be confusing and very painful. When you open your heart to love someone, your heart is at the mercy of that relationship. When we define love only from our experiences with other adults, we can get stuck in the pain of loving. If we have been hurt or let down as an adult or child, this causes us to close our heart in order to protect ourselves. How are we supposed to understand the true nature of love when we mix in all the complications of relationships?

If our purpose is to learn to love on both gross and subtle levels, we have to learn first that a closed heart is scared and does not want to trust love. Instead of trying to understand how and why we were hurt, we should change our focus to trying to understand and connect to love.

About eight years ago my ex-husband and I separated and eventually divorced. Of course it was difficult to let go of the relationship because I had expected our marriage to last. I knew my heart was broken, and I was very aware that I was closing it so that I would never feel that same hurt again. I'm not for a moment saying that I was the only one from that marriage who felt pain. I'm just stating what I went through. It took time and effort to open my heart and not feel pain. I remember talking to a fellow yoga class student about trying to focus on my heart area and feel love. I explained to her that it felt like I had built a brick wall around my heart. She was able to relate to what I was saying because she was going through a marriage breakup herself. It was comforting to be understood, but I knew that I was the only one who would be able to break through that wall.

I tried to stay away from thoughts about "the hows and whys" of the hurt and instead took my attention to my heart area and imagined love. I used images I've seen in nature and sounds of music I love to help me connect to a universal love. Universal love, love in its purest form, is always there for us even when we come to it with a broken or closed heart.

A new definition of love should be developed so that we know where to go when we are stuck in the confusion and pain of life and relationships. If we are made of the same stuff as the universe (love), then connection to this, consciously choosing to connect, brings us our true power, universal power. Our biggest responsibility and our biggest challenge is to stay connected to universal love. If we keep moving in the direction of love, we know we are on the right path.

We can think of love as a universal force that runs through everything and our connection to this love as our spiritual evolution. Universal love gives us the place or feeling of absolute strength. It is the source of guidance for which we yearn. It is where we must always turn and how we must strive to be. Love is the answer. It is always that simple. No matter where we are, what we are doing, or how confused we are, we have to know that our answers come from our source - the love of the universe. When we wonder where to go, we must remember that love is our purpose. Making a connection to this pure love and trying to maintain this connection is our purpose.

So, how do we make this connection? How do we maintain it, and what breaks this connection? These are the real questions of life. Our spiritual evolution depends on us exploring and answering these questions. Each chapter in "Changing Focus" examines different ways in which we break our connection to love. Our lack of understanding about how the two modes of our brain function is at the root of most of our misperceptions of the true reality of love. By becoming aware of how to shift our focus from left brain thinking to right brain processing, we allow ourselves to see the love based, more subtle and profound side of our situation. The next three chapters explore the right mode and left mode and discuss them in the context of creative processing and logical thinking. Using that as a foundation, the rest of the book covers common practices and thoughts of our daily living that cause us to break the connection to love and suggests thoughts and methods for reconnection to love.

When we try to find peace by first looking at the problem, we are moving in the wrong direction. The truest answers come from love. When we connect to love first, we are then ready to have our questions answered. The source of love and our connection to this source always comes first. That is why I titled the book "Changing Focus". We are so often focused on the problems and need to learn that focusing on love is what solves the problems. We can change our focus from fear to love, from the outside world to the inside world, from logic to imagination and creative thinking, from our physical material existence to spiritual energy, and from loneliness to feeling connected to and part of the love of the universe.

When we realize that we are often focusing on the wrong thing, we have a very powerful tool to assist us in our spiritual growth. If love is our purpose, then the main goal of our life should be to refine our understanding of how and where we should focus our mind and energy so that we can increase our connection to love. This is a process, and a complete understanding of how to stay connected to love requires time.

I use subtle beauties of life from nature, art, and music to become more and more aware of and absorbed in universal love. I also use yoga to relax my body and to become aware of subtle energy and emotions. It is much easier to relax your mind and get rid of negative thoughts and emotions if you breathe slowly and deeply and try to let your physical body relax. I also sit by the window or outside and stare at the colors and shapes of the plants and trees in my yard. After a busy day, this calms me down and helps me let go of the day's events. When I sing and dance with my children, I am almost immediately able to enter a frame of mind that sees the bigger picture of life. Like all of these activities, it helps me to feel universal love and to remember that I am part of a universal plan.

When we define, discover, feel, and use love at increasingly subtle levels, we become more and more convinced of the necessity of staying focused on love and learn ways to maintain and strengthen this connection.

What is profound love, the love that creates and is our spirit and unites us with the purpose of everything in existence? It takes time to know, but we can experience some of it through prayer or meditation. When we pray, our goal is to connect to God or love. If we pray effectively and consistently, we can develop a bond to love. Through time this bond to love strengthens, and we become more effective as decision makers. Love becomes our guidance mechanism and our source of energy and inner peace. If our daily connection to love, or prayer time, is strong, we automatically carry the love we've gained with us after we've finished praying. The love we carry brings energy and clarity of mind and helps us choose thoughts and actions that keep us in tune with love. When we don't pray effectively or regularly enough, it is difficult to make a strong connection to love. I try to follow a list of priorities I've set for myself that help me maintain my connection to love. At the top of that list is daily meditation. I used to think that there had to be a set amount of time for my meditation, but I've come to realize that 15 minutes can work as effectively as one hour. It depends on how well I can focus on that particular day. When I skip a few days or a week, I can really sense that I am off balance. At those times I don't feel strong, and my feelings of being alone in the universe begin to increase.

When I first turned towards the universe for guidance, it was difficult for me to feel heard or to sense that I am loved by the universe. When I concentrated on building a relationship with love through effective praying, I learned how to feel heard, understood, supported, and guided by universal love. We can approach prayer and connection to love the same way we would approach love in our relationships with other people. If we know how to love and be loved by other people, we realize that really listening, understanding, and supporting are the foundation of a loving relationship. Although some of us have never been taught how to have strong relationship skills, we don't need to worry because connecting with the love of the universe is easier than connecting with people. We know that universal love can be completely trusted, and this makes it much easier for us to feel completely heard, understood, and supported. When we try to open our heart to pray, we may still carry the left brain logic that tells us that it does not make sense to trust love, and it does not seem logical to pray, but if we imagine and step beyond the disbelief and uncertainty into trust, we can begin to make the connection. Prayer involves imagining we are able to trust the love of the universe, imagining we are completely heard, understood, and supported, and imagining we will be guided. Imagining the connection carries you into making the connection. Prayer also involves feeling thankful to something so powerful and wonderful. When you feel gratitude towards universal love, you increase your connection to it and open your heart. Gradually, we are able to feel more love, and with this comes the certainty, the belief and knowing that we are loved. So, in order to step beyond the pain of human love and the logic of our left brain thinking, we must imagine and feel gratitude. Creative thought or right mode perception is a key to connecting to love in prayer. Increasing our respect for and understanding of imagination and the creative right brain is closely tied to understanding and connecting to universal love and our spiritual evolution.

Connection to love during prayer is very intense. It brings with it a peaceful feeling in the body and a joyfulness in the heart. Love also quiets our fears and clears our mind of controlled thought and replaces them with insights and answers to questions we have about our life. Prayer is a very powerful thing when you learn to do it effectively. It is like a school. When we finish we carry the knowledge and experience it gave us back to our daily lives. It is the cornerstone of spiritual evolution because it is the time when we absolutely know the love of the universe. Effective prayer allows us to trust and know love in its purest form. I didn't always pray effectively. I was able to relax my body, but my mind would wander. Most of my growth in prayer occurred during the first year after my marriage ended. Feeling the pain in my heart gave me the incentive to focus on my heart and replace the pain with love. It took a while to learn to trust that universal love is always there for me, but the more I imagined it and the more gratitude I felt, the greater I trusted and lived in love. Even now, if I am going through some challenge in my life, I can forget to focus on love. I know now though, through experience, that praying effectively is always where I must turn.

As we evolve in our understanding of love through prayer, we are able to maintain a stronger connection to it at all times. We connect to it during our daily experiences and learn that we have a love based guidance center within us that is meant to be used. The guidance center is in our heart area and comes in the form of inner knowing or instincts.

I used to find the word instincts difficult to explain or define. I just knew that certain things felt right and that I had used this sense of rightness very consciously while making major decisions in my life. Without question, the most life impacting decision I have ever made occurred when I was 18 years old. At that time I found out I was pregnant. This was a turning point in my life. Having to face the prospect of marriage and raising a child at such a young age was extremely overwhelming for me. I was confused about love and didn't feel ready to get married. In the late 70's most people considered that being a single parent was not an option for a young woman. If you became pregnant, you gave your child up for adoption or got married. I knew that I had some incredibly important decisions to make, and I didn't want to make the wrong choice. I also knew, even though I was very young, that I had to choose what felt right for me. I spent a lot of time trying to get closer and closer to what felt right. I spent many hours alone trying to clear my mind and eventually realized that I could not get married and that I had to raise my child on my own. I did do those things and have always been certain that I made the right choice. My instincts were guiding me then and have guided me through many other big decisions I have had to make over the years. It wasn't until I became more clear about the right brain and left brain and refined my meditation practices that I came to realize that instincts create a frame of mind that we can stay tapped into during daily living.

Our instincts or guidance center is directly tied to universal love, and the more directly we contact universal love in prayer the closer we come to knowing our guidance center. Our heart opens in prayer, and this opening cuts away the pain and hurt that keeps us from trusting and sensing our instincts. It is obvious that we can't spend our entire day in silent prayer, so we are given an internal guidance mechanism to refer to at all times. Every moment we are faced with decisions, and every moment we should be moving with what feels right according to our guidance center. We should be following our instincts, going with the flow of what feels right, or going with the flow of love. During every conversation and every series of thoughts and actions, we have the choice of doing what feels right in terms of staying connected to or following the guidance of love. This probably sounds complicated, but it becomes a state of mind. It becomes effortless.

Following our instincts from moment to moment is just making sure our choices don't cause us to fall out of line with our feelings of peace and love. Doing the right action or being in a love state at all times is what we are aiming to do. This comes with practice, but it feels magical when you can have an entire day where you felt connected to and guided by universal love. Ultimately, WE are choosing to follow the guidance center, but it feels like our choices are being given to us. The day flows without conflict from within, and we are certain that we are moving in the right direction.

Using meditation or prayer and trying to follow our internal guidance mechanism are two powerful ways we can connect to love. Our daily existence offers us many other opportunities to perceive love and to get to know it in more subtle forms. The way we approach situations, how we interpret what we encounter, what we think about, how we think, what we choose to focus on, all of these things give us opportunities to perceive love in many different forms. Love is our purpose, and searching for love is our mission.

CHAPTER 2
Right Brain/Left Brain

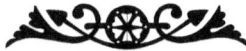

O ur purpose is to love, to constantly be aware of and feel the presence of love. "Changing Focus" is about the process of staying connected to love. I am introducing a tool that can be used to assist us in trying to stay focused on love. The tool is left brain/right brain awareness and learning to shift from the left mode to the right mode of processing information or perceiving reality. This chapter is a discussion of the two modes of the brain. I introduce them and define them based on my experiences as an artist, teacher, and student. I recommend that you read "Drawing on the Right Side of the Brain" by Dr. Betty Edwards to learn more about how our brain halves function.

Before I read "Drawing on the Right Side of the Brain", I knew very little about right brain/left brain. I didn't know that my brain was capable of holding me back from controlling my perceptions of life. The book was given to me by an artist friend. At the time I was wanting to pursue painting as a career and was trying to learn as much as I could about being an artist. My friend had no idea how much this book meant to me. To her it was a book that taught a drawing method. To me it was a book that revealed an approach to life. I was so excited about the larger life answers it gave me that I wanted to discuss these ideas with her and another artist. I ended up realizing that I had to develop these ideas on my own. It ended up taking a lot more time than I had expected, but my instincts told me to keep going, so that is what I did.

What we think controls our emotions. What we think and feel usually governs our actions. How we act sets our future. We have to turn back to what we think and how we think by examining how each brain half works. Our spiritual evolution should include a study of the dual nature of human thinking and perceiving.

Before science really studied the two hemispheres of the brain, it was thought that the right hemisphere (R-mode) was less evolved or capable than the left hemisphere (L-mode). Since then, we have come to realize that it is not a matter of one being more capable than the other. They are just different. They are designed to do different tasks.

The R-mode, most commonly referred to as our creative side, processes what it absorbs through a creative method. When it is being used it allows us to be inventive, intuitive, imaginative, nonverbal, visual, and to exist in a time-free mode. When we are in R-mode we are fascinated by, appreciate, and become absorbed in complexity, details, and subtleties that L-mode is not interested in experiencing. R-mode allows our senses to become fully stimulated so we can see, smell, hear, taste, and feel things we normally wouldn't notice. We slow down, our mind clears, our fears diminish, our body relaxes, and we breathe more deeply when we are fully engaged in R-mode. When in this state we lessen our tendencies towards judgment and attachment and increase our feelings of certainty and confidence.

I experienced this state very intensely as a child and teenager during our summers at the cottage. Back then there were very few people living in that particular area, so we could go for days without seeing anybody outside of our family. We had no television there, so we were outdoors most of the time. To many people, especially in this day and age, this would seem like a boring situation, but if you know how to immerse yourself in nature it becomes an incredible adventure. When I was tired of playing with my brothers and sisters, I would go off alone for hours. I went exploring. I would stop and look at everything that had an interesting design, or texture, or color, etc.. Some of my most vivid memories are of times I spent sitting alone for hours on a favorite rock that is partially surrounded by the ocean. I would watch everything I could see underneath the ocean's surface and also be entranced by the waves hitting the rocks, shells, and seaweed. I smelled the air and touched all of the fascinating textures. The longer I sat there the more interested I became in the experience. I didn't want to leave. I felt so calm and satisfied. My body and mind were completely relaxed. Obviously, these hours and days helped me to tune into the subtle patterns and details of nature, but, more significantly, I was learning how to be fully engaged in R-mode.

I am sure all of us can think of activities in our lives that bring us into this type of state. When I list all of the qualities of R-mode, it makes it seem complicated, but every one of us experiences it in some form or other. In order to help you identify more clearly with the R-mode state, I'll use some examples. Have you ever been walking on a beach or in the woods and found yourself becoming more alert and more relaxed and comfortable? Probably you slowed down your pace and decided to "stop and smell the roses". Well, if you examine these activities more closely, I'm sure you will find that you were experiencing a lot of the R-mode qualities I just listed. Maybe your busy thoughts and worries left your mind, and you were left with a feeling of contentment. You may have begun to notice the details of the beauty around you like the smell of the air, the sounds of nature, the details of beautiful shapes and colors in rocks, trees, flowers, weeds, bark, etc.. R-mode looks for beauty because it absorbs it and appreciates it on its most subtle level. Maybe you felt less of a need to talk and were content to be in the moment. Insights and clarity about something may have come to you, and you had a gut level feeling of certainty and confidence about the rightness of the insight. I'm sure an experience like this would end with the shock at how much time had passed. Of course we can have varying degrees of intensity of an experience like this, but the point to recognize is that you were in an R-mode based state of mind.

A more simple exercise in using R-mode could be taking the time to eat something slowly so that you can fully enjoy its flavors and smells. Close your eyes, slow down, relax, and really enjoy the food. Don't think, just let yourself become absorbed in the subtleties of the flavors and textures, etc.. As I said, this is a more simple or less intense R-mode experience. It does not involve being profoundly touched or using all or most of the R-mode qualities, but it is using R-mode. When you can use R-mode in something as simple as eating, you realize that you can use it to enhance many different experiences. It is a way of approaching something-a process of slowing down and fully engaging in what you are doing. It is something we are completely capable of doing. Most likely, we have never tried to point it out to ourselves before.

The strategy for gaining access to R-mode is to present the brain with a job that L-mode will turn down. So, what is L-mode, and what jobs will it turn down? L-mode is analytical, logical, rational, and likes to verbalize or use language. It is the part of our brain that wants to organize and plan things using step by step logic. In writing this book, I had to plan and write the logical sequence of my points. In order to explain the conclusions I had drawn, I had to build on a series of logical ideas. At first, what I had written explained the facts of my thesis but that was all it had done. The manuscript lacked a personalized and emotionally engaging element. This was pointed out to me by an editor who read a portion of my manuscript, and it made perfect sense to me. My logical thinking had taken over too much of my writing, so I added more R-mode expression and color to the facts.

L-mode sees situations as jobs. It is the mechanical part of our thinking. Because of this, efficiency is a priority. It keeps track of time and likes to be in control. Its most powerful quality is judgment. It likes to compare things and judge them based on what it knows logically. It does this by using stored information and symbols that are simplified versions of the original image or experience. The logic based style of L-mode keeps challenging us to think logically. If we step away from what we know as fact, L-mode tells us we are not being realistic. How many times does logic and being too quick to judge get in the way of us following something more abstract and subtle like instincts? How can a mind that spends most of its time planning, organizing, analyzing, and thinking rationally expect to instantly or easily open up to creative thoughts and experiences? L-mode is in command of our brain processing most of the time because we live in a language and technological based culture and because of its nature. The nature of L-mode is to be efficient, so it does not like it when we slow down. The nature of L-mode is to be verbal, so it doesn't like it when we stop thinking and talking. Its nature is to rationalize, judge, and analyze, so it enjoys all of the thinking we do when we are trying to figure things out in our mind. Because our education systems teach mainly L-mode subjects with L-mode methods and do not favor or, in some cases, even support teaching R-mode methods or subjects, our culture encourages an L-mode approach to life. I'm sure all of us can relate to feeling driven by a need to be organized, rational, logical, etc.. It's not that we shouldn't have and develop these qualities, it's just that we are in that mode so much of the time and can't seem to get away from it easily.

Discussion of the right and left hemispheres is not common, so most people don't realize that they have the power to slow down and lessen the intensity of their logical mind. It is possible to do this, and it is extremely useful to do this. Too much time spent in L-mode exhausts us and leaves us feeling unfulfilled. It keeps us stuck in many ways.

In answer to the second part of the question "What is L-mode, and what jobs will it turn down?", L-mode will turn down things designed for R-mode. As you read along in the book, you will come to a more clear understanding of R-mode and the different tasks for which it is designed. It has taken years for me to broaden my understanding of the creative mind. The more I learn about the dual nature of my mind, the more ways I notice I can apply this information to my daily life. When I was younger I existed without this information and suffered unnecessarily. I remember feeling extremely overwhelmed by life when I was in my early 20's. I was a single parent attending university trying to survive and create a financially stable future for my son and myself. It would have helped me out so much if I had had this information back then. Instead of feeling overwhelmed and vulnerable, I would have known how to protect and rejuvenate myself. My attitude towards life was completely colored by the sense that all I could count on to change my situation was hard work and dedication to my responsibilities. This of course is a big part of freeing yourself but protecting and preserving an empowered attitude makes the journey much more bearable. Now I take breaks to assess my attitude. I give myself sense stimulating experiences in nature. I focus on subtle feelings of love and try to expand them. I relax my mind when I'm thinking too much about things, and I try to move at a slow pace so that I can extract the beauty from situations. This slow pace and sensitivity to subtle beauties is R-mode. I know this now. So, when I become overwhelmed, I know that I must turn off the mechanical approach. I trust that I have the power and methods to change my mode of perception.

Because L-mode is so aggressive, it often overpowers R-mode. How often do we listen to ourselves when we know we are being too hard on ourselves, thinking too much, or moving at a fast pace for too long? We know how powerful these drives are from many experiences we've had. We can learn how to make the shift from L-mode to R-mode. First, we have to set up conditions that cause us to make the shift. Then, with experience, it becomes easier to consciously control the shift.

It becomes easier, for example, to listen when we tell ourselves that we are being overly analytical.

Our challenge is to become more aware of each mode and then learn how to set up the right conditions to make the shift. I will give two examples of conditions you can set up when you draw. These conditions encourage R-mode to take over. These examples are based on exercises from the drawing method developed by Dr. Betty Edwards. Even if you don't like to draw, you should do these exercises because they provide really good examples of the R-mode shift. One exercise you can do is turn a very simple cartoon style drawing you want to copy upside-down. Draw the upside-down image of a person or table, etc.. Even though the upside-down image looks like lines and shapes, not a person or table, draw it anyway. Draw the shapes and lines. Don't try to name or identify what you see as an upside-down arm or table leg. Try to become absorbed in seeing what is there rather than identifying symbols. Earlier in the chapter I said that L-mode uses stored information and symbols that are simplified versions of the original image or experience. L-mode is based in efficiency. It tries to organize and store data so that it can use it later to assist it with analytical and logical thinking. R-mode, on the other hand, takes things as they are in the present moment. It experiences the uniqueness and newness of things rather than using stored symbols. For the sake of efficiency, L-mode stores simplified versions of things, especially complex visual images. So, our L-mode symbol for a person probably resembles a stick man or a young child's drawing of a person. Unless you update or revise these simplified stored L-mode symbols through R-mode observation, L-mode is only capable of drawing stored symbols that do not look like realistic visual images. That is why so many people think they can't draw. They try to draw, L-mode takes charge, and it pulls up a simplified version or symbol of what they are drawing. You end up drawing what you "think" is in front of you or your symbol for the figures or objects in front of you instead of drawing what is actually there. If you concentrate on seeing and drawing shapes and lines rather than letting L-mode name and identify the parts of the picture, R-mode will take over. Do this exercise and observe any R-mode responses. Take note of feeling engrossed in the act of drawing, losing a sense of time, being fascinated by what you see, etc..

When you look at a picture of a person, or chair, or any realistic picture upside-down, L-mode can't make sense of it. It asks, "What is it? I don't recognize it, so it's not important, and I'm not interested in drawing it. It's just a bunch of lines and shapes." L-mode finds it difficult to place the abstract shapes into a category. Remember, L-mode sees in terms of stored symbols. If it looks at something and can't figure out what it is based on its file of stored symbols, it loses interest in it and is willing to let R-mode take over the task of drawing. R-mode, on the other hand, loves visual detail. It doesn't care what the picture is or whether it is recognizable. It just wants to examine the detail. It is thrilled to look at subtle line movements, subtle variations in shape and contour, and every shade of darkness and light. The more complex the lines and shadows, the more interesting the task becomes to R-mode. Once R-mode is in charge it draws what is there, not what it thinks is there. R-mode sees and draws the unique details of the picture, and L-mode does not see or draw unique, new details. It draws what it "thinks" is there based on stored, simplified images.

If you have no experience with drawing, this example may seem inappropriate or difficult to understand, but trust me when I tell you that it is a very useful way of getting to know the differences between L-mode and R-mode. Stick with me.

Another condition you can set up to encourage R-mode to take over is to do a pure contour drawing. Pure contour drawing is drawing the edges or lines of a complex form or image without taking your eyes off the complex image. If you choose to draw your thumb, don't bend it so that you will be able to see more lines. Stare at a line on your thumb and follow it with your eyes. Move your eyes AS SLOWLY AS POSSIBLE trying to see absolutely every bend, curve, and connecting line that's there. At the same time, you draw with your other hand, moving the pencil at exactly the same speed and with exactly the same movements as your eyes. Don't look at your pencil or what it's producing. Keep your eyes totally focused on your thumb. The more detail you see and the more slowly you move, the greater your chances of making the shift from L-mode to R-mode. The point of the exercise is to make the shift so don't worry about whether the drawing is realistic. After you've been looking and drawing for a few minutes, you will probably begin to become more and more fascinated with the detail of the lines you see. Maybe you will take a few deep breaths and feel relaxed. If you move your eyes and pencil slowly enough and do the exercise for 10 minutes or so (set a timer), you will make the shift from L-mode to R-mode. Try the exercise so that you can experience the shift and write down what you felt like after you became fascinated by the details of the lines.

This type of drawing exercise is the most effective one you could use to make the shift from L-mode to R-mode because you are not looking at what your pencil is producing; therefore, the L-mode critic can't criticize what you are drawing. It can, however, tell you that the exercise is stupid, but try to not listen. The L-mode critic is powerful, and when we listen to the criticism in our mind about what we are drawing, we are still in L-mode. Fighting the critic in our mind is the artist's biggest challenge. It is also one of our biggest challenges in daily life. The critic keeps us stuck. The best thing to do is to learn about how to make the shift from L-mode to R-mode. Move from being overly self-critical to being calm and relaxed and enjoying the feeling of observing what you are experiencing in the moment.

You may be wondering what these drawing examples have to do with spiritual growth. They are very important lessons to understand because they are directly tied to understanding the shift from L-mode to R-mode. They each give a very real example that shows that the shift is possible. When you learn to make the shift, you realize that the shift can be used in many daily situations, even if it is as simple as shifting from L-mode to R-mode because you want to calm down and relax. When doing the upside-down drawing, L-mode turns off as long as you see the drawing as unnameable shapes rather than a leg, a hand, etc.. During the pure contour drawing, L-mode shuts off once you become absorbed in the complexity of the lines you see. L-mode does not find the complexity of subtle movements in lines an interesting thing, so it gives the task to R-mode. So, here we have two ways of making the shift. We can give L-mode something it does not recognize from stored symbols or something that requires moving slowly and being fascinated with subtle changes and detail. How can we relate these examples to life and spiritual awareness and growth? First, spiritual growth requires learning to see love as the essence of everything. Staying connected to the same old view, being narrow-minded, or reacting to what we THINK is there are all L-mode ways of perceiving a situation. What if we stopped using stored "symbols" of experience and viewed with an open-minded approach? Second, what if we tried to be in the moment by using a slow paced approach, learning to become aware of the subtle details in our lives? If we are stuck with stored views and quick responses, how are we going to see love as the essence of all of life and the foundation for spiritual growth?

The more I apply these two techniques to my life, the more I realize how severely I had held myself back in the past. Although I was strong in terms of self-discipline and making difficult choices, I have often felt distressed and controlled by my life. It has only been in the past five years or so, since I have better understood these right brain techniques and have applied them to more situations, that I feel more in charge of my life. Now I know that being open-minded is a choice you can make while viewing anything and so is moving slowly and seeing the beauty in subtle details. Being hopeless or narrow-minded about certain things does not have to be a permanent character trait. When you apply the skill of opening your mind to viewing what's actually there, rather than responding from stored experiences, you will likely be able to understand the purpose of what you are facing.

I have always been comfortable with opening myself to new situations. I have been willing to step away from traditional views. I am not what you would call an obvious nonconformist, but I am definitely a nonconformist in many ways. I am certain that a large part of this attitude was developed because of having been exposed to nature and creativity, but another influence was the "hippy" mentality. Back in the early and mid 70's, there was a major influx of hippies to our area. They came mainly from the U.S. and were attracted to our area because of political issues and the lightly populated, natural ocean setting. It is difficult to describe the impact these young adults had on our community, but it was intense. Our region was occupied primarily by conservative Scottish Catholics. The university and hospital were partially run by the church, and our ties to our Scottish ancestry were strong. The mentality contrast between us and our new neighbors could not have been more contrasting. On a daily basis we were shocked by their "free" behavior. They were very visible. They stood out and didn't ask for permission to be themselves. They were nonconformists. They did things based on what felt right for them. Eventually, they became a valued part of our community. They taught many of us to see, first hand, what it means to live a daily existence with a very open mind. Making their own mistakes, as everyone does, they still provided a valuable example that we can learn from. They tried to experience a life with great depth. They respected the environment. They ate natural foods and lived in natural settings. They valued the arts and spoke about peace and equality. They embraced a slow pace and looked at life from a new perspective.

I was encouraged to use an open-minded, slow paced approach to my life by a wide variety of sources. Now, I can look back at these influences to help me better understand the L-mode R-mode shift. But, the easiest way to first recognize the shift is to experience it while doing the drawing exercises I've described in this chapter.

Teaching drawing is about teaching people to see and draw what is there, not what they "think" is there. You have to draw the shapes in front of you, not what you've stored as a symbol for what you are drawing. The shift becomes clear in drawing when you realize that seeing is the key. Learning to see, to look very closely at what is in front of you is a skill very few of us have been taught. I'm not trying to teach you how to become an accomplished artist. I just want you to realize that we usually look at things with L-mode (what we think they are), and this is very different than seeing them from an R-mode perspective (as they really exist at the present moment).

Let's look back at the examples I gave earlier. If you went for that same walk along the beach or in the woods with an L-mode frame of mind, you would have been in a rush and would not have noticed or enjoyed all of the beauty around you. Of course you would have realized that you were passing trees or rocks, etc., but they would not have seemed really interesting or worth stopping for for closer observation. Instead of fully engaging in the experience, your mind would have been unable to stop chattering, and your thoughts would have consumed your experience. Even though you were surrounded by the peace and calmness of nature, you would not have sensed it, seen it, or absorbed it. The peace or love of an experience is always there. We just have to learn how to slow down, open our mind, and focus on the newness and subtle beauty of the experience.

The other example I gave of R-mode involved eating. An R-mode method of eating is slow and attention is given to the subtle smells, textures, tastes, etc.. L-mode eating is fast and efficient with very little attention being paid to enjoying the food. L-mode looks at food as an experience of necessity. We are hungry or anxious, etc., and we have to satisfy these cravings. L-mode is logical and efficient about this experience it knows so well. Through experience from eating, we know that a potato or a chip is what it is, and it may taste good but L-mode says, "I've done that before, and I don't need to experience it again. Let's just get it done quickly and efficiently.". So many experiences have more to offer when we approach them through R-mode.

I definitely don't want you to obsess on every experience you have, trying to figure out the mode you are in but being aware of the modes is very useful. Becoming aware of R-mode and L-mode and how to shift from one to the other is a useful tool. We can use it to help us understand life and to increase our awareness of love.

CHAPTER 3

Creativity

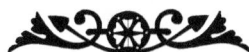

ow many people think about creativity or try to use it as a process for guiding their lives? In the previous chapter, I spoke about the differences between L-mode and R-mode. From the examples I gave, you can see that L-mode and R-mode are very different modes of processing situations and life. L-mode is based in logic and judgment, and R-mode is based in a creative, in the moment approach. If we are in L-mode most of the time, which most of us are, how are we going to experience creativity? How are we going to learn about the creative process and use it to enhance our experiences in life? The reason we don't discuss and study the creative process and understand our creative nature is because learning to appreciate creativity requires a shift to R-mode awareness. You have to open your mind, slow down, and experience R-mode before you will understand the value of creativity. Since most of us rarely slow down enough to experience this shift, society does not discuss creativity, and most of us have a limited understanding of its potential value in our lives. This chapter is an attempt to broaden our views of creativity.

How does creativity relate to art? Art can be seen as an activity requiring imagination and skill used to create works of art. It is both the process of creating the work and the work itself. There is the art of painting and the work of art which is the painting. There is a process and a product or end result of that process of the artist. This distinction between process and product is important to note. It points out the fact that there are two different ways of viewing art. Most of the time, we think of art as a product, a piece of music, a movie, a book, or a drawing when we should be looking as closely or more closely at art as a process. This is where creativity enters the picture. Creativity is a process, not a product, but when most of us think of creativity we think of art and the products of art. Since most people do not consider themselves to be artists, they draw the conclusion that they must not be creative. This point is so important to understand. If you think that you have to be an artist, one who is able to produce works of art, in order to be creative, where does that leave your interest in learning about creativity? If you believe that you are not creative, based on the fact that you have no or little background in "the arts", why would you want to spend time trying to increase your understanding of creativity? Society uses the terms "creative thinking" and "imagination", but the depth of these ideas is not really examined or understood by most people. For the most part, the topic of creativity is left for artists, others not taking part because they don't consider themselves artistically inclined.

We don't understand creativity, and we also find creativity a bit intimidating because of its association with art. In fact, even among artists the creative process is not really understood. It is almost considered to be a mystery. We can look at it with disinterest, intimidation, or confusion, but the fact remains that the process of creativity is mainly an R-mode process. Everyone has a creative right brain or an R-mode way of viewing, and everyone should feel comfortable knowing that they are meant to be creative. In order to live up to our full potential, we need to use our creative right brain. We have great untapped potential that is easy to access, we just have to pay attention to the R-mode way.

What keeps us away from creativity, and how do we benefit from keeping in touch with creativity? For me, my living environment plays a big role in keeping me in touch with my creative self. I have found that the more in touch I am with my creative self, the more I approach life as a creative process. (I will discuss the creative process later.) I have created an environment in and around my home that helps me to remember to slow down. I have done this mainly through the use of nature and a simple or uncluttered home. My home used to have more "stuff" than I needed. Gradually, I have eliminated many unnecessary items and am left with a more peaceful living space. Once I did this, I found it a lot easier to relax while in my home. I was encouraged to meditate or to do some quiet reflecting. This new situation helped me maintain a creative attitude. Now, I am more easily able to look at my experiences and daily challenges as being part of a process of growth because I am less distracted. I use nature to help me stay calm. I plant flowers. I sit outside and appreciate everything around me. I listen to nature's sounds and smell its smells. The more often I give myself experiences that include a slow pace and an uncluttered living space, the easier it is for me to have a creative or R-mode attitude and to remember that life is a creative process. As time goes by, I have become less afraid of life's challenges and more accepting of the idea that everything that happens fits, in some way. I am encouraging myself to trust my creative attitude.

The average person comes from a school system and a society of L-mode training. We have not been trained to be creative, and to trust creativity. We have been trained and are being trained to be efficient, logical, and analytical planners. From very early on in life, we see that life requires logic, discipline, and hard work. All of these qualities are extremely valuable and absolutely necessary and desirable, but they are not the only qualities and skills that we should be teaching ourselves and our children. What happens to us when we value all of our L-mode skills to a point where we don't even know how to slow down and relax? What are we teaching ourselves about the deeper meaning of our lives? What is guiding us and helping us put all of the pieces together? When financial survival is met solely from hard work and no play, our lives are empty. It may be difficult to imagine anything but working at a fast pace, but it is necessary because our children are learning from our example. When we look at what is happening in North American schools, we see that the creative arts are very low on the list of priorities. They are the first thing that comes to many people's minds when financial cuts are required in the school system. I know that in North America there is an undercurrent of objection to "the arts" cuts in the school systems. Every once in a while, over the past few years, I have heard celebrities and artists speak out about how important it is to put the creative arts back into our schools. As a teacher in Nova Scotia, I am very aware of the lack of understanding our government and the general public has had about the value of "the arts". Recently, some Canadian provinces have re-established these programs after having cut them out almost completely, but I sense that most people consider these programs to be less important than "real" subjects. The point that these people are not getting is that creative arts programs give our children a well rounded education. With well designed music, drama, dance, and art programs, our children will develop their ability to see and hear subtleties they would normally overlook. They will become better observers and will learn to appreciate slowing down. Our school systems encourage logical, analytical thinking and teach our children to be efficient and organized. Children also need to learn to slow down and be calm and to be open-minded and nonjudgmental during their day at school. The current situation in our school systems is indicative of how little we understand and therefore value our creative mind. The part of us that slows down and enjoys the moment is way too silent because of lack of use. If we want to begin to feel more depth and meaning in daily life, and if we want to learn to engage in life as a creative process, we have to use our time and money to explore and develop our sensitive, imaginative, and creative selves.

Creativity is not a luxury or a gift given to only a few. Creativity is meant to be used as a way of viewing life and its experiences. Through the lens of the creative mind, we can be guided through life with peaceful emotions and inspirational insights. This is a right we have, not something we should ignore. It is as much a part of us as our logical mind, but gaining access to it requires turning down our logical mind. Try to imagine a long-term plan for your life that includes a commitment to trying to see without controlling and fearing new situations. What if you were able to engage in a lifelong mission of decreasing fear of money, death, loneliness, etc., and you knew for certain that you were on the right path. The only requirements would be that you continued to study and use your right brain, you expanded your understanding of love, and you viewed your life as a creative process? Instead of running through that forest or along that beach I described in the previous chapter, you learned to walk along in R-mode. An R-mode way of perceiving a walk can be used as an opportunity to learn about how to engage in life as a creative process. Life is meant to be felt, experienced, and enjoyed. It is a creative process, not a planned, step-by-step race aimed at the final result or product. Life is not about the end of the race, the win. It is the entire run (walk). The enjoyment of life comes from understanding and engaging in the process, not from an exhaustive, competitive race that propels us towards a desired product.

I have noticed, as I am sure many of you have, that many children of this generation seem to be much less connected to natural stimuli than we were at their age. I can remember my childhood friends being playful and busy, but I don't remember them having the ADD type symptoms that I currently see in so many of today's children. Part of their behavior is in response to having been greatly stimulated by our technological world, but figuring out where and how this change occurred should not remove us from giving our children helpful growth experiences that pull them away from this busy mentality. What I have found that works really well with my children is to allow them to express themselves freely when they are playing. I encourage them to dance, sing, and dress up in ways they want to, and I watch them perform. I also make sure their lives are not too busy, and I encourage them to explore the outdoors. They calm down and become centered during these free expression and nature explorations.

Children seem to be thinking and moving at too fast a pace. This is a societal habit. Almost all of us have been moving at too fast a pace for too long. We can encourage ourselves and our children to step out of the race by allowing them and ourselves to do activities that slow us down and cause us to see the beauty and feel the peace and delight in what we are doing. By doing this, we are teaching ourselves and training our children to become students of the creative process of life. Small R-mode experiences end up teaching us to be strong and free and to flow with life's ups and downs.

A process can be orderly and established, but it can also be a series of steps resulting from natural or heartfelt actions producing gradual growth and change. How can we expect to grow and increase our understanding of and sense of fulfillment towards life unless we are feeling our way along, unless we approach life as a creative process? When you think that life is about getting or working towards happiness at the expense of your health, relationships with your family, etc., you are forgetting that you have an intuitive, sensitive, feeling side that needs to be guiding you. Our commitment to growing in our understanding of the creative R-mode side of ourselves is what sets the process of creative living in motion. We can't understand at the beginning of the process how creative living is possible, but that is the nature of creativity. In order to experience it you must first trust it. If we trust creativity, we can gradually come to know why life has to be viewed as a creative process.

When you observe what is required to create a work of art, you can conclude that life lessons can be learned from the process it took to create that work. Looking directly at a work of art can inspire many wonderful emotions and thoughts, but the act of creating is something all of us should try to understand. When you begin to create something, you are driven by an urge to begin. The beginning is very often done over time and often inspired unexpectedly. You may get a vague idea of something you feel compelled to create, but it usually remains vague until you let it brew in your mind for days, or maybe months, or years. This brewing time can be both exciting and confusing. You know that something is being worked on in your mind, in almost a subconscious way, but when you try to fit it all together, it does not make sense. The whole picture does not piece together. You don't want to get your hopes up for fear that your idea is not worth developing, but, at the same time, you can't give up. Part of you knows that at some point, things will become more clear, and you will eventually be able to consciously pull forward a beginning or developed idea. The secret is allowing it the time it needs to develop. Trying to judge it too soon, or trying to force it into a mold before it is ready, delays the process by increasing your level of frustration. Sit back (so to speak), and wait until you KNOW (instinctive knowing) that it is time to begin the painting, writing, music, etc.. When you begin the physical act of writing, etc., you have to remember, once again, that you can't judge what you are doing too often or too severely. When you over judge, you tend to stop the flow of inspiration. This same rule applies until the completion of the project. Trying to become less of a judge and more instinct guided is always the goal. When you begin to create, your instincts will be quiet, but they will let you know with great certainty where you should step next. If you are in touch with a guidance system, your instincts, or inner knowing, you sense when something doesn't work and when something does work. The tricky part is making sure you follow your instincts rather than your L-mode critic. Usually, your indication that your instincts are speaking is that what occurs to you comes with calmness rather than panic. The next thing that you must remember is that you have to trust more than control. Trusting that it will work out o.k. allows you to keep going. It keeps you from labeling your abilities and your work worthless. Trusting also keeps your mind and imagination open. The opposite to trusting is trying to control the outcome to a point where you are afraid that everything is not perfect, so you move painfully or quit. When you try to control, it has to be done in moderation and be aimed mainly at things like form and structure. (The medium you are working in dictates a lot about what needs to be controlled.) The control issue has its biggest power over our confidence. If you are creating something, your thoughts can tell you many negative reasons why what you are doing does not make sense, etc.. When you push these thoughts aside by getting into the beauty of what you are doing and follow the guidance from your instincts, you are learning to trust. This is when open-mindedness, new ideas, inspiration, and clarity about the work are revealed.

This process of suspending judgment during the brewing time, giving your work time to develop, trusting your instincts and not pushing, learning to trust rather than control the process, searching for the beauty, experiencing the use of imagination and the inspiration of an open, clear, insightful mind is the creative process. The end result, what you create, is a whole different side of art. The art we need to learn about is the creative process of art.

If you take these same lessons you've learned from the creative process of creating art and apply them to life, you see the importance of these skills. How often have we been encouraged to experience the qualities of suspending judgment, accepting that some things need time to brew or form on their own, and to let go of trying to control situations in order to learn the benefits that come from trusting what our instincts tell us to trust? I'm sure that there are many people who have had lessons in their lives that have taught them to use these skills, but examining the process of creating a work of art is an easier way to teach those lessons. The lessons from creating in "the arts" are there as a gift to help us learn absolutely essential lessons for life. Math, the sciences, and technology can, on some advanced levels, require the experiences of creativity, but for the most part, the arts work as the most effective and accessible medium for teaching us about creativity and the creative process.

If we compare what is going on during the creative process in art to how the two modes of the brain correspond with this, we will see that the creative process in art or life requires mainly an R-mode approach. Suspending judgment is a powerful R-mode quality. It is probably the most powerful part of R-mode in terms of it being able to turn off L-mode. L-mode wants to judge, categorize, and fit things into stored symbols of experience. All of this goes totally against a more creative approach of letting things take their own course. L-mode wants to push things forward, to be efficient. It is very aware of the passage of time, and if it thinks that time is being wasted or too much time has gone by, it really pushes you to think negatively about what you are doing. Control is to L-mode what trust is to R-mode.

When writing or drawing, I find it really easy to notice the negative L-mode thoughts I have that push me to speed up and to not move intuitively. I find it much more difficult to notice my negative L-mode becoming too strong while I am going about my daily life. I am like most people. My life can be really busy. Even though I am getting much better at pacing myself, I can catch myself trying to run through the day so that I can get everything done. I'm certain that I will continue to have busy days, so my approach to each day will have to continue to become more intuitive. The more I trust my intuition, the more I realize that L-mode thoughts and pacing don't have to control my behavior and attitude. I am frequently shocked at how controlling L-mode can be and how free I feel when I trust my instincts and let things fall into place.

The connection to imagination, insight, inspiration, and clarity of mind during the creative process is definitely R-mode based. These qualities, or skills, are what we normally think of when we think of creating a work of art. What needs to be noticed here is that not only are these skills for artistic creation, but they are skills that can be applied to our approach to life. While I am writing, I try to stay calm. I know that I have to focus on opening myself to an R-mode frame of mind. Even if I am writing the logical sequence of my ideas and need to use the organizational skills of L-mode, I still need R-mode for inspiration and clarity, etc.. I take the time to relax and expect to have insightful thoughts and inspiration. I try to imagine that what I want to accomplish is already accomplished. Gradually, I have trained myself to do this during tension-filled or overwhelming situations in my daily life. I am always seeing new ways to apply these skills. I find that they work really well when dealing with people and situations that test my patience. If I am in a hurry and am standing in line at a store, I imagine that everything will work out. I change my attitude from panic and a need to control the situation to one of going with the flow. I used to get uptight in those types of situations and that would cause me to feel controlled by them. Most times, I end up noticing that as soon as I imagine I can trust that things will work out, I see that the situation does not have to control my emotions in a negative way. Another thing I do is use my imagination to disengage from a confrontation. If I am having a discussion with someone, and I realize that both of us are becoming frustrated, I stop talking and imagine that I am calm. I trust that things will fall into place, even if my point is not made or heard. I clear my mind and let go of my need to control the situation. Usually, I hear what the other person is saying in a new way, and I am able to figure out how to diffuse the conversation. L-mode wants to control the thoughts I have, but I can allow my imagination to step forward by becoming objective and trusting my instincts. These are skills that can be learned, but L-mode discourages us from valuing or developing these skills. L-mode does not like the non-judgmental, trusting part of creativity and will fight, with thoughts and negative feelings, to have us stop being creative. It is its function to do and be as it was structured to do and be. It does a great job at what it does, but we have to let R-mode in, and we have to become comfortable with what R-mode does. We CAN learn the skills of trust, inspirational thinking, letting go and being in the moment, open-mindedness, and so many more things. The resource is there. We just need to learn more about R-mode and its connection to the creative process.

The creative process is our evolutionary process. It relates directly to the art of "being" or living with uncertainty and trusting our intuition and the organization of the universe. When we look at the creative process this way, we are able to tie it to our spiritual development.

It is our tendency to feel victimized by devastation created by something or someone we can't control, but we remain victims when we keep that attitude. The creative process teaches us that what we want to create comes through, only if it is meant to and that it comes about more easily after we let go of a need to control the speed and direction of the process. We must trust that our intuition and inspiration will guide us in the right direction. What I take away from devastating situations is to look at them as opportunity to remember to release fear and control and to embrace trust. I choose to turn the situations in to an experience that aid in my spiritual evolution by remembering that life is a creative process that requires me to trust the process and the organization of the universe. With a world full of uncertainty and confusing presentations, the only answer is to trust the universe and the creative process.

Learning to trust the universe, or our abstract reality, makes that reality more real. Learning to trust our spiritual essence, our intuitive guidance, love, a universal plan, requires letting go of a logical perception of reality and living within a creative process of spiritual growth. We need to learn about our entire nature, not just the mechanical, product producing methods we've been using. The art of living can be learned, and we can expect our creative experiences in life to enhance our feeling of connection to ourselves and the guidance and love of the universe. No matter what or where we are, the answers come from our source, the love of the universe. Making a connection and maintaining this connection to love is our purpose, and the most effective way to get there is by learning how to approach life as a creative process. As I have said, the creative process is our evolutionary process.

The R-mode qualities we need to be paying attention to are imagination, intuition, noticing and experiencing the subtleties of something rather than thinking about it, creative thinking, trusting the process, giving room for new perceptions, holding back on judgment, etc.. We have examined these and more qualities in the example I gave in this chapter on creating a work of art and the examples I gave in the previous chapter on drawing, taking a walk, or eating in R-mode. In order to understand these R-mode qualities and turn them into skills, we can examine simple experiences we have had in our own lives. We can look at how often we think of using an R-mode type of approach and how often we choose an L-mode approach. If we can recall a situation or thought we have had, and try to imagine how differently we would have felt about it if we had approached it with, for example, trust rather than control, I'm sure the value of this practice will be made obvious. Try to spend some time comparing how situations or thoughts would have turned out or how they would have made you feel if you had turned off L-mode and shifted to R-mode.

Try to turn a situation upside-down, so to speak, by looking at it from a new perspective. Keep in mind the following points: R-mode likes to look at a situation or thing as it is, in the moment. L-mode tends to put things into categories and makes reference to them from stored symbols rather than seeing them for what they are in their own unique form and in the present moment. R-mode sees the newness and is fascinated by the details, complexity, and beauty of this newness while L-mode loses interest in what it doesn't recognize. It likes to analyze and categorize. R-mode moves slowly and enjoys the experience while L-mode likes to move quickly and efficiently. R-mode likes to use thought in the form of insights and imagination, and L-mode prefers logical thinking. R-mode is content to let things brew and doesn't have a time schedule or expectation of perfection, and L-mode thinks brewing an idea makes that idea useless. L-mode judges based on efficiency and logic and what is in accordance with its stored logical standards. If we are in L-mode for most of the time and have based our view of life on this type of thinking, what type of nagging thoughts do we have to fight off continuously? If we look at life as a gradual learning process, valuing uncertainty and trusting the process, we experience life as it is meant to be experienced. But, if we are constantly judging our lives, ourselves, others, etc. based on a close-minded, efficiency based, strictly logical frame of mind, chances are uncertainty fills us with fearful thoughts and trusting the guidance of the universe is difficult for us to know.

L-mode keeps us stuck in the step-by-step logic of life. It wants products and concrete results. The finished product and things that go according to plan are most valued by L-mode. Whether you are approaching a drawing, creating a work of art, eating, going for a walk, or viewing life, L-mode and R-mode are capable of producing very different results. Both are necessary ways of viewing, but R-mode is not used or understood enough.

When we think of creativity, we should know that it is a process that can be applied to the act of creating a work of art, the biggest work of art being our lives.

"Changing Focus" is meant to encourage people to slow down and open their minds to seeing life from more of a creative perspective. Life is meant to be fully experienced, and R-mode gives us tools to help us feel and absorb life more completely and to move with the subtle messages and mysteries of life. Changing your focus from a logical to a creative, instinct guided approach will increase your feeling of certainty that your life has a purpose and that you are connected to a force that governs everything. Isn't that the point of spiritual evolution? Aren't we meant to continuously increase our feeling of connectedness to the universe? Let's step back from task oriented, fast paced, money driven motives often enough to enjoy the benefits and pleasures of living with creativity.

CHAPTER 4

L-Mode Thinking

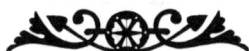

W hat is L-mode thinking? Basically, this is the most important question in the book in the sense that examining and understanding our thinking is the cornerstone to understanding and knowing ourselves.

When we examine the creative process, we realize that R-mode dominates this process, but this does not mean that L-mode is totally cast aside during the creative process. L-mode gives us clarity about what we produce, it's just a different kind of clarity than the clear thought we get from instincts or intuition. L-mode clarity comes from logic. In most situations, we need logic to help us understand things. For example, if you read this book and none of it made logical sense, you wouldn't be able to absorb the messages I'm trying to get across to you. If you were feeling inspired and were having a conversation with someone, and your thoughts were not following a logical pattern, you would not be able to express yourself clearly. Even though R-mode and L-mode seem to be independent from each other, they very often have to work together. In writing a book, you have to use the creative process as well as set up a logical outline and sequence of thoughts. In having an inspired discussion, you need both logic and creative inspiration. The reason I'm mentioning this is because this chapter focuses on L-mode thinking. I don't want to confuse you by implying that L-mode thinking and R-mode are totally separate from each other. It's not that simple. A lot of it depends on the type of L-mode or R-mode function you are engaged in and the intensity with which you are engaged. The point is not that you strive to know exactly how and to what extent you are using each mode but to develop R-mode skills that are useful and decrease L-mode ways that are harmful. I do not claim to know precisely how, at every moment, and during every activity and thought each brain half is functioning. I am pointing out general tendencies of each mode to help you become more aware of the fact that two modes exist. This does not mean that one must be completely dormant in order for the other to be active. If you are doing an R-mode task, that does not necessarily mean that L-mode is completely dormant or uninvolved in that task. It just means that R-mode is more dominant at that moment.

The reason this chapter is about L-mode thinking is because L-mode loves to think. When you consider that we are using this mode most of the time, we should examine how it tends to think. What is L-mode thinking? It is thinking based in logic, analysis, planning, organizing, judging, categorizing, and other left brain ways. Imagine how many thoughts that includes.

One of the more major discoveries I've made while exploring L-mode thinking is how closely tied we are to judgment. I used to watch myself jump to conclusions about people, myself, or situations, figuring that logically these things deserved to be judged. When I study these same types of things now, I consider that maybe judgment can be released. Probably because of being raised in a traditional Catholic home and community, I tended to be very hard on myself. Although I would fight to do what felt right for me, I would often be fighting off nagging thoughts of self-criticism. When you think about it, we can view any situation as one of growth. It's true that we may have to pay a price for mistakes we've made, but judging oneself and others too harshly is an unnecessary habit. L-mode works that way. It views us (people), our actions, and our personal vulnerabilities with the idea that these things have to be judged. This overly critical way is a habit, one that needs to be broken. When we realize that judgment is just a mode we are in, we can choose to make it less necessary. I don't always have to know if I like this or that or if this or that is logically right or wrong. I can just BE and exist where and as I am. I often switch modes by slowing down and focusing on beauty in all of its subtle forms. By removing judgment, I leave room for seeing beauty.

How many of our daily thoughts are based in L-mode functions? How often do we examine the way we are thinking or what we are thinking? These are huge questions. It may seem a bit extreme to be examining thought so closely, but we are thinking most of the time. We live in a verbal culture. We communicate through so many technological mediums and get so much information to think about that we are rarely encouraged to examine or take a break from our thoughts. R-mode doesn't approach thought in the same way as L-mode. R-mode does not like to think too much. It would rather be absorbed in the task at hand and stay open to inspiration or instinctive, intuitive type thoughts. The distinction between these two ways of approaching thought is what is needed to be understood by society. The left brain likes to control situations and understand them completely and immediately. The creative mind wants to experience things in as many emotionally calming and sense engaging ways as possible. It is sort of like the difference between a hunter and a naturalist. L-mode attacks problems or inconsistencies in order to solve them as a hunter would hunt for the purpose of getting game. He may approach the hunt with great skill and awareness of his surroundings, but his mission has one purpose which is to hit his target. A naturalist could walk the same route through the woods as the hunter, but his purpose is to experience the walk, not to walk until he finds the specific thing for which he is searching. I try to approach my day with as much of an engaging attitude as possible. I usually have a number of goals that I need to accomplish, but I try to stay open to experiencing each moment. I use a combination of the two modes of perception but really try to be in the moment rather than being too goal oriented. It ends up feeling like I am being led through my day and to my goals rather than feeling like I spent the day trying to control and accomplish things.

There is such a big difference between the two modes of thinking, and it is rarely discussed. We are thinking with L-mode most of the time and, for the most part, we don't realize we have another option. It's not that logical and rational type thinking is wrong, it's not, but when you are in the habit of being verbal and thinking analytically most of the time, the tendency is to become controlled by your thinking. Too much L-mode thinking can cause controlling, overly critical, and obsessive type thinking. How often do we catch ourselves worrying, being fearful, thinking negatively, or feeling hopeless and unable to break out of those thoughts? All of us know what it feels like to let our anxieties and fears take over our thoughts. Everyone has difficulties and uncertainties to face each day, but some days we are stronger than we are on other days. Why is that? How are we able to stop or lessen our anxiety on some days and not on others? A big part of this is being able or unable to turn off the L-mode chatter. This allows us to stop thinking long enough to feel a connection to something bigger. We can quit trying to control the situation and instead relax and stop thinking about the problem. When we replace a need to control and to have logical, instant solutions to our worries with the R-mode way of relaxing and waiting for guidance and inspiration, we have tapped into a tremendously powerful tool or skill.

R-mode sees how things exist over time. It tries to look at the whole picture. It doesn't think with controlled thinking. Instead it relies on insights, intuition, imagination, and going with gut feelings. It goes with thoughts that feel right or true and ones that make you feel peaceful. Our senses can be used as a tool to aid us in turning off our L-mode thoughts. They allow you to notice and become fascinated by subtle details. You can slow your pace and turn down L-mode thinking by noticing and absorbing beauty through your senses. When I do this, I feel in touch with my instincts. I get a sense of truth that hits me at a gut level. Also, I don't feel compelled to analyze and judge. I enjoy the experience I am in and feel it rather than think about it too much. R-mode prefers not to think and speak too much. It prefers experience over thinking about the experience. L-mode creates the constant chatter in our mind. It loves to be working quickly, doing what it thinks is useful. Action, activity, and a fast pace feed this mentality. Even when the problem is not able to be solved right away, it keeps thinking about it. It does not like to slow down thinking, even when the thoughts are negative.

Feeling panic and fear are the extreme forms of too much negative L-mode thinking. We have to learn how to quiet its chatter and to increase peaceful and positive R-mode thoughts. So
often there has been something going on in my life that bothers
me or needs a solution, and a solution is not available. I used to
remain disturbed by those things. Now I can justify forgetting
about them and ask the universe to provide a solution. I give
myself time away from the issue by refusing to think about the
issue. My financial situation, like most people's, can swing to
low points. Not knowing how I will make ends meet has, in the
past, had a debilitating effect on me. I could get so wrapped up
in trying to solve the problem that my thoughts would be non-
stop. This would bring me to a state of despair. When I learned
that I didn't have to keep playing the scenario over and over in
my mind with over-analysis based on a need for a logical outcomes, I was freeing myself. I now know that L-mode tries to
force a solution, but a solution is not always immediately available. Thinking over what may happen based on all of the available information can often lead to a realization that there is no
plausible solution. R-mode can let me release the need to control the outcome and frees me to stay in the moment and enjoy
my life. No matter how hard it is to stop myself from trying to
control things, I always try to because I now know the power of
R-mode. Not only does it help me become more peaceful and
relaxed, it helps me to get in touch with my instincts which give
me messages that offer me solutions. I am not giving up power
by releasing L-mode chatter, I am gaining strength from my
internal guidance system.

Here is another example of the chatter of L-mode thinking.
I have to pay close attention to the thoughts I am having when

I am working on a drawing or a painting. My mind can think things like, "This drawing doesn't look good. I can't make it look realistic. I don't know how to create something beautiful or worthwhile.", etc.. It's not so much that L-mode is trying to think negatively, it just wants to think and be practical and efficient all of the time. The criticism arises because the work is not complete. It will look realistic and beautiful if I give it time. Even if it is not a masterpiece, why should I allow my thoughts to keep me from trying and learning from my efforts. Over time, your L-mode learns that R-mode can draw, so these insecure thoughts become less strong. But, even though I know I can produce realistic drawings, I still have to watch for too much L-mode chatter. When I'm not having an easy or enjoyable time with the drawing, I examine what I'm thinking. Usually, just the act of examining the thoughts is enough to turn them off. I can also concentrate on the complexity and beauty of the details and know that this will cause L-mode thinking to decrease.

For a new artist or someone drawing for the first time, your L-mode will chatter away with reasons why you should hurry, or stop, or recognize that your drawing is not perfect, or that you have no talent, etc.. It can be so overwhelming that it really does discourage you from trying. L-mode chatter can be very convincing, and it feels very real. It really does make you feel insecure. The secret is to know that it does not have to control you. A good example of this is something that has occurred over and over with me, especially when I was first learning to paint. I would be in R-mode or working calmly, feeling inspired and confident, and then gradually, I would begin to examine my work with a critical eye. I would begin to tear it apart by thinking about how terrible it looked. I would consider scraping all the paint off and starting all over again. Of course, in some cases, this is a good decision, but sometimes it is just L-mode getting in the way. In many cases, it is being overly judgmental. Very often I would find that leaving the painting alone for a few days would allow me to come back with a fresher or less judgmental perspective. In many cases, I would go back to the painting and see that what I had criticized a day or two earlier was in fact the most beautiful part of the painting. I would be shocked by the contrast between my two different interpretations of the exact same section of a painting. One attitude was so negative and unable to see the beauty, and the other was inspired, positive, peaceful, and comforted by the beauty. My mind was seeing one section of my painting in two completely different ways. So, over time, I've learned when to step away from a work in order to allow myself to see it from a new perspective. Instead of letting L-mode chatter control my actions, I walk away until the chatter loosens its grip. Sometimes we can get L-mode thinking to turn off by giving ourselves time away from the issue. Other times we have to replace the chatter with inspired thinking. The chatter of L-mode is powerful, and turning off L-mode thoughts that are too negative requires practice. It requires knowing that we don't have to be controlled by the negative thinking. Using a logical or critical eye is a way of perceiving something, but it is not the only way. L-mode does not like to give up control, but it will if we remember that we have a choice. We choose what we think. We can choose to imagine, to feel inspired, to see life as a creative process, to stop being overly critical towards life and ourselves, etc.. A lot of our fears and negative feelings are based on how we perceive things. Perception is based on how we think and what we think. If we carry our rational, analytic, and logic- based thinking with us constantly, our perceptions will be based on those types of thoughts. If we develop an ability to see the big picture and to use more intuition and less rational thinking, our perceptions will be more expansive.

L-mode chatter could be described as thinking too much. A good example of this chattering is when your mind is constantly thinking about the past and future. R-mode, for the most part, stays in the present. It is an in the moment way of experiencing things. When you are worried or are thinking repetitively about what already happened and/or what may happen, you are think-ing too much. You have to realize that too much of this type of chatter in our minds leaves us feeling disconnected from the present. It is the same with thoughts about situations we are currently undergoing. When we keep running them through our mind, we are not experiencing what is happening in the moment. We are thinking about our lives more than we are experiencing our lives. This is not to say that we should value only R-mode. We just need to know how and when to turn L-mode thinking off. When L-mode chatter turns into controlling and obsessive thinking, it is negative. It is removing us from the peace in our mind and heart. Our goal is to feel love and peace.

Right now, as I'm writing this chapter, I have to fight off L-mode chatter. I need to use L-mode to sequence my thoughts and write with logical sense, but at the same time, I have to let go of logic in order to allow the writing to come from inspira-tion. This is a challenge and something that takes patience and time to learn. It is so easy to get stuck, in writing or in daily life, when we forget to let go of logic and certainty. On any given day, we can find ourselves trying to know the logical progression or the end result of something before the project is complete. How can I know, with absolute certainty, that what I am writing will make sense to others, that I will be satisfied with it, that it will be logical and inspirational, or that it will have value and be valued? How do I know for sure that I will be able to verbalize what I want to express in this chapter? If I spend too much time thinking about having to know the end result and how to accomplish this in a logical way, I will lose my inspiration. I will be removing the creative ingredient, the part that pulls it all together or gives you a way of describing something that fits perfectly. These gifts of inspiration and guidance seem to come out of thin air, but they do exist for us to use. You block yourself from receiving them if you try to logically control, or know beforehand, everything you create. When you stop being overly judgmental and analytical with your thinking about what you are working on, you open the door to receiving new possibilities. Too much judgment or analysis, etc. turns into L-mode chatter. It usually comes in small repetitive thoughts, but they are powerful.

I can't emphasize enough how important it is to become aware of how often we are facing L-mode chatter. It comes in different forms, some more negative than others, but it exists too dominantly in our thinking as individuals and as a society. I have seen so many television shows debate and analyze a situation or person to a point of great extremes. Many things can be deemed "newsworthy" and then be observed with intense scrutiny and judgment. People tend to not want to let go of "good story". We are so easily able to lock into L-mode obsessive-analysis that shows like this are successful. Also, I have observed many conversations that direct attention further and further into this type of analysis. Looking at these types of shows and conversations as "L-mode feeders" makes them seem less interesting.

Thinking with too much judgment and control, or fearing the past and future are L-mode thoughts. These thought patterns seem like they are organized into negative and positive thinking, with too much L-mode being negative thought and R-mode producing positive thoughts. This is definitely not true. L-mode does and can encourage tremendously important and powerfully positive thinking, but letting L-mode run loose in chatter gives it plenty of opportunity to spend too much time analyzing anything that crosses our mind. L-mode chatter can tend to narrow our thinking down to repetitive, controlling thoughts. R-mode is by nature expansive, open-minded, non-judgmental, in the moment, and creative. So chances are, when you are using R-mode, your thoughts will tend to be positive. You will have fewer thoughts, and generally they will come from a feeling of acceptance and inspiration.

I'm sure most of us are very used to hearing about positive and negative attitudes, but how or when have we been taught about the two ways of our brain. Knowing about the brain can give us more control over our thinking. Instead of feeling like we have to accept that it is too difficult to stay positive, we can work instead on developing the skill of turning off L-mode chatter. It's much easier to change what you think when you know how the brain halves process information. The exact same situation can be viewed very differently simply by shifting from one mode to the other. This takes away the belief that we are controlled by our thoughts. We don't have to let L-mode dominate, and we do this, in part, by realizing that L-mode exists.

It is easy to understand and accept R-mode when it comes to drawing and the creative process. These creative acts seem separate from what society views as "real life", so labeling them as requiring a special way of processing information is easy to accept. The difficulty comes when we try to identify with R-mode and L-mode in terms of daily life and thinking. We have been living with L-mode in charge for so long that R-mode or creativity doesn't seem to be necessary or even real in anything except art. We know that creativity exists, but it has a time and place. Logic dictates this thought, and the only way around it is to try to open up your mind to the possibility that we have to learn to think differently. Society accepts things based on our discoveries, so we can change what is accepted if we discover new things. Our L-mode type of viewing will accept new information about R-mode and creativity when the new information becomes real, something we know from experience. We need proof from experience to satisfy our logical thinking. We need to experience a creative way in "real life" so that we believe it when we tell ourselves that we have to stop being so logical.

I know this is sounding complex, but it is an overpowering barrier to break through. The thinking mind we use most of the time is L-mode and because of the way it functions, it has created a barrier for us to experiencing any other way. We think and behave according to L-mode, and when we are faced with the idea that we need to let go, we, or our L-mode thoughts, become more dominant and logical and opposed to letting go. We can quiet its chatter and decrease its dominance simply by recognizing that it exists, but we can't stop there. We have to constantly remind ourselves that L-mode likes to be in charge. It will not let us give up thinking logically unless we learn more and more about how it functions.

Logically, I should lead my life sticking to well thought through plans, but uncertainty is necessary if we want to follow guidance from the Universe. We have to surrender part of our comfort if we want to follow a path that resonates with the universal plan. L-mode wants certainty. It wants to know what to expect and it wants to control the outcome. It has taken me a number of years to put R-mode in charge of this concept and to put this into action in my life. I find I am still noticing how desperately I want to control certain outcomes, but they have become fewer. Here is an example of a response I've worked to change. I'm sure most parents can relate to having a strong need to guide their children, usually with too much control, as their children make decisions that will affect their upcoming adult life. It is so difficult to let go and give teenagers and young adults the freedom and respect they require by allowing them to make their own choices and mistakes. It took me a couple of years to let my children have their freedom, but I've realized that uncertainty, in some situations, is our only choice. We can't control all or many outcomes with thoughts or plans. Even though our logical mind finds this idea very difficult to understand, it is true.

We have to begin to notice how we think. We don't need to be obsessive about this task, but persistence is required. Our thoughts are not our identity, so we can rise above our logic and L-mode chatter and still exist. This is what I call being an "objective observer". The following may sound like a silly thing to say, but letting go of a long-held method of thinking can be very powerful. We are capable of identifying very deeply with our thoughts, so changing our thought patterns may make us feel as though we are letting go of part of our identity. The perception we create of "who we are" is based on how we perceive ourselves and our surrounding. It is our perception that we are changing, not our identity. It is part of life to change and grow, so we don't have to be fearful of this change, even if it feels big.

The idea that we have no or very little public education or understanding of the power and control of L-mode thinking, and the idea that we are just beginning to learn about such a fundamental part of our nature is shocking. How could we have evolved to this point and not known that our mode or method of thinking and perception is something we can choose? How could we have missed this? Well, actually, many older cultures base their spiritual practices in meditation or quieting the mind. The idea that too much logic, analysis, and judgment remove you from experiencing the moment is not new. We don't have widespread discussion and education about the importance of quieting the mind. Now that we are able to discuss this mind chatter and mode of perception in the context of R-mode and L-mode, we have a more concrete way of understanding this duality.

When we examine thinking, we can look at the small, moment to moment, thoughts that run through our mind (many times almost unnoticed), and we can look at the bigger thoughts, or general perceptions, that we have about our goals, lives, families, and our beliefs, etc.. The small thoughts may be running through our mind noticed, but if they go unnoticed, I'm sure we would be shocked at how many times we repeat thoughts that should not be repeated. When we are working on something that needs to be thought through, we can use as much analysis and judgment as necessary. This could apply to something as simple as scheduling errands or something as complex as designing a building. Repetition and careful analysis are necessary for those tasks. The more careful, controlled, and deliberate the thoughts, the more effective the results. On the other hand, we may be trying to solve a problem we are facing and, after careful examination, we either can't see a solution or don't know if there is a solution. Either way, we know we want to stop thinking about it because it is taking our attention away from being totally engaged in the moment. It can exist in our mind on a conscious level, but often it repeats itself over and over again without us realizing that we are thinking about it. The danger in this is that it affects our mood and attitude during the day and it keeps us distracted from fully experiencing life. L-mode finds it difficult to relinquish control. If we are having a thought that we do not want to have, how can we remove it from our mind? L-mode wants to analyze and rethink the problem until it is solved. Many times, the solution is not possible or the thoughts are simply fear based worries about the future and/or past. Do we want to keep rethinking things that cause us to feel fear and distract us from being totally involved in living in the moment? Sometimes we want thoughts to be mulling around in our mind. Also, often we need to be doing more than one thing at once, and sometimes our creative mind requires free floating thinking. But when we have unwanted, repetitive thoughts that we remain fully or partially focused on, we need to know how to let them go. They become a distraction to us even when we don't stay completely focused on them. They keep running through our mind, often leading to a set pattern we've developed over the years.

The first step we must take is that we become aware that our L-mode is working overtime. It is chattering when we have unwanted, repetitive thoughts. They could fear based, or simply uninteresting. We can stop the chatter by choosing to engage more fully in the details and beauty of the moment. It's just like the examples I described in the drawing exercises. When we slow down and focus on the details of the present and search for beauty, we lock into being in the moment. Obviously this is something that requires practice, but negative chatter from L-mode will stop when we turn to an R-mode state of being focused on the beauty of the moment.

I know this is not easy to do, but with practice it becomes easier. If you are in a negative L-mode frame of mind, first you need to spend some time trying to calm down. You could take some deep breaths and try to relax your body. After you have put your attention on relaxing, then you can begin to concentrate on what is going on in your mind. If you remember that you don't have to keep thinking L-mode thoughts over and over, you can begin to replace the chatter with being present in the moment. Remember the walk I described in the second chapter where being in R-mode allowed you to slow down, to breathe more deeply, to sigh and relax, to be fascinated by and notice subtle beauties, and to have inspired, more expansive thoughts? Use this as a model. All of us have had experiences like this one, even if they came to us unexpectedly. We can choose to be in R-mode. We don't have to wait for it to happen to us. If you use the R-mode experiences you've had as a reference, you will find that relating to R-mode is possible. Try to feel connected to a slower pace, and let go of the sense of urgency in your thinking. Consciously pay attention to your gut feelings or instincts. Imagine peace and look for insights rather than controlled, repetitive thoughts. Try to minimize thoughts and keep them directed towards beauty, love, suspended judgment, appreciation, and acceptance of what must be accepted. This does not mean that you will give up thinking about something that needs to be resolved. You just need a break from the chatter. If you are judging, analyzing, or trying to control things to a point where your thinking affects you negatively, turning off the chatter must be your priority. When you think about your family, your job, your responsibilities towards yourself and others, financial concerns, trying to complete a work of art, etc., you have a choice about how you approach these thoughts. If you remember you have this choice, you can begin to decrease the tendency to overuse L-mode thinking.

In my search for easier and more efficient ways to connect to R-mode, when L-mode thinking is negatively distracting me, I have discovered that having a daily time of conscious and deliberate connection to universal love really helps. Every day I spend time calming myself down. Some days it's for 15 minutes and other days it's for 1 ½ hours. I clear my mind by trying to feel connected to love. The trick I've learned is to try to reach the point where you can really imagine you are loved by the universe. When you imagine you are completely heard, understood, and supported by the universe, you are able to turn L-mode off almost completely. You lock into a feeling of love, certainty, and strength, and you know that guidance is always with you. When I do this every day, when I am able to make this connection and sustain it for a while, expanded and insightful R-mode thinking occurs and remains with me after I have finished this exercise. It often gives me solutions to issues that are troubling me, and it always provides a break from too much L-mode chatter. If I lose sight of where and how my thoughts should be focused during the day, I always get back to inspired, open-minded thinking when I practice a direct connection to imagining and knowing that I am loved by the universe. I call this meditation, but in effect, I am turning off L-mode and focusing on love. So, when my mind is racing with too many analytical or fear based thoughts of the future and past, etc., I depend on the residual benefits of my prayer time and my increasing awareness of how to replace L-mode chatter with R-mode being. These experiences encourage me to look for the beauty in the moment and to know that it's o.k. to stop L-mode thinking sometimes. When I am thinking with L-mode too much, it is because L-mode likes to think, not because it has to think.

When thinking about larger life questions such as our purpose and the meaning of life, R-mode allows us to see the big picture through inspired, intuitive thoughts. R-mode perception doesn't have to have logical proof to understand spiritual unity with the universe. It allows us to place ourselves in the experience of this other reality. It gives us the opportunity to have expanded, open-minded thoughts, and this is what carries us to the subtle realm. When we know and feel the subtle presence of the universe, we are experiencing it through R-mode perception. When we intellectually understand and discuss the force of the universe, L-mode perception is dominant. L-mode would question the logic of our connection to the universe or try to control, analyze, or organize the experience, while R-mode would just exist in it. R-mode encourages us to exist in the moment. It allows us to BE, to accept, and to not judge. The essence of R-mode is experience. It gives us tools to BE or a way of being in the fullness of the experience rather than thinking about the experience. You are able to have certainty of the existence of a universal plan and force when you are fully experiencing the universal force. If you forget the experience and feel pain and confusion about the uncertainty and seemingly unfairness of life, you are thinking too much. You have to turn off your L-mode based thoughts and instead experience feelings of connection to the love of the universe. Stop the logic and chatter and experience the love.

Thinking about daily life concerns, or thinking about our purpose and the meaning of life requires thought. We need to have logical, controlled, efficient, analytical, systematic, organized, and judgment based L-mode thoughts. But, when we think about and process daily and larger life issues with too much of this type of thinking, we can become controlled by our thinking. We should not be thinking with L-mode all of the time. We have to know how to turn it off when it is too dominant. A break from L-mode logic and chatter is necessary in order to be fully present in the moment and to more fully experience and understand the subtle reality of life.

CHAPTER 5

The Subtle Reality of Existence

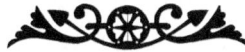

We experience the obvious reality of life every day. We have responsibilities, aspirations and dreams, relationships, feelings, thoughts, and experiences that create our reality. Most of the time, our daily existence feels like the only reality, but what if we could see each moment through a lens of love? What if everything we experienced was connected to a sense of purpose and unity with the universe? Then we would be experiencing our life in a new reality. What we now experience as reality would become part of a bigger system.

I was trained from a young age to separate spirit from daily life. Just the act of going to church, once a week, used to make Sundays seem like a holy day. Sundays felt special, but I was unable to transfer that same feeling to the other days of the week. Sitting in church on Sundays, at Christmas Mass, and on other holy church days was powerful for me as a child. These experiences trained me to put God and spirit into a special time and place. I'm sure many people are able to get past that sort of spirit isolation, but my young mind couldn't think that expansively. To me, God was living in church and expected us to come and visit him once a week. The Priest would make sure we received a message from God, and we were to take the weekly message home and try to apply it to our lives. Most times I would not really get the main point of what the Priest had said, so I found it difficult to remember anything. In fact, I would forget about God most days. I did say prayers at home some times, but they were so drilled into my mind that their message was lost and detached from God or spirit. My daily reality was separate from conscious spirit awareness for my entire young life. It wasn't until I was in my late teens and early twenties that I expanded my notion or definition of God or spirit. It began with the discovery of other religions and spiritual practices. Because of my study and practice of meditation, Eastern Philosophies, and yoga, my notion of spirit expanded to become more of a personal, moment to moment reality. Now I try to remember my spirit to a point where it feels like my identity, and I try to connect my daily existence to the universe.

So often, we see our lives as being separate from the purpose of the universe. For example, how does taking out the garbage or buying groceries connect to anything like spiritual evolution and the unified force of love? When you see your daily actions and thoughts as "real life", and feel connected to a universal plan at specific times, you are experiencing life as a reality separate from universal love. There is a way of having a constant connection to love and the purpose of the universe. This may sound confusing, but our "real life", or daily existence, is meant to be lived with a constant awareness of spirit or love. It is possible to exist where we exist and yet know that every moment is connected to a system that guides us and the universe.

You may be wondering why I am trying to make this distinction between what we perceive as reality and what is meant to be perceived as reality. Well, we are caught up in "real life" almost all of the time, and "real life", for the most part, does not include the constant certainty of universal guidance and love. Try to imagine what life would be like if you always felt guided by and connected to the most loving and peaceful feelings you have ever felt. During times of crisis and prayer, we often feel these types of feelings because of an intense need to connect to something larger than ourselves. When we connect to love, we know that we are where we should be. The connection feels right, and it gives us insights and strength to deal with our lives. What we have to teach ourselves is that this connection can be felt every day. We can strive to have a constant connection to the strength and guidance of the universe.

Sometime, when I meditate or pray, I aim for a sense of connection to loving beings or guides so that I can more easily feel heard and supported. By approaching prayer in this way, I am creating a more realatible relationship with the subtle realm. Instead of thinking of the subtle realm as something abstract and separate from me, I try to think of it as something more personally connected to me and my life.

Our logical mind becomes more and more convinced that "real life" is separate from the experience of universal love unless we encourage ourselves to move away from this mentality. We have to turn away from many established ways of being and viewing life in order to reach a place where life offers constant subtle, yet powerful, messages of love and support. When we begin to shift our emphasis from "real life" thoughts and experiences to staying connected to the subtle reality of love, our "real life" enters the subtle realm. Our situation is the same, but our perception of our situation changes. One really simple, but powerful, idea I've learned is to change my view of the passage of time. I have often been so tied to meeting goals and getting through a day, that I create a busy frame of mind in myself and forget that I am not moving slowly enough to be in the moment. I have figured out that this busy way of being is partially based on being on a linear time schedule. We look at birth as the beginning and death as the end and all the things that occur in the middle as events that run along a time line. We progress in age and learning from year to year, and we accomplish what we believe we need to accomplish, always hoping that we will move closer towards peace and stability. This is such a linear approach. It makes me feel like I am always reaching for something in front of me. Linear time can be seen as an illusion. We can make progressions without feeling trapped by a time line. When I remind myself that everything in this moment is as it is meant to be, I stop trying to control outcomes, and I slow down my pace. I try to release the notion that time is passing so that I don't push myself too hard and forget my spirit and the subtle realm.

When we perceive life with an awareness of and connection to the subtle realm, we stop trying to control our lives and instead move with our lives. We free our mind from over judgment, over analysis, and fear based L-mode thinking. We are able to receive inspiration and support from following the guidance of love based thoughts and perceptions. The subtle reality is "real life" immersed in love-based perception. When we look for love, ask for guidance from the universe, trust the guidance, and act in accordance with the messages we receive, our daily lives may stay the same, but our frame of mind elevates us to a state of peace. We see everything through a lens of insight, wisdom, peace, certainty, and unity. The subtle reality exists in our mind in the sense that we can connect to it and live in it by changing how we perceive "real life". When we break away from the notion that "real life" is separate from the spiritual realm, we begin to live our daily lives within the subtle realm.

We have to learn to change our focus from "real life" to the subtle reality. There are so many things in life that capture our attention to a point where we lose a sense of spiritual purpose and guidance. The daily experiences of going to work, paying bills, taking care of ourselves and our families, looking forward to vacations, accomplishing goals, relaxing, watching television, doing household chores, etc. occupy most of our time and thoughts. It is not very often that we think we have time to slow down or a choice about cutting back on our responsibilities. This leaves us in a situation where we feel like we are constantly working at just trying to keep up with everything. When you search for a subtle reality in this type of "real life" situation, first you have to slow down and give yourself time to understand how to change your focus. A fast pace will keep you engaged in a fast paced mentality. If you want to know and unite with the subtle reality of love, you need to slow down first. Moving at a fast pace and being organized requires L-mode thinking. You need logical and analytical thinking in order to plan, structure, and organize what you want to accomplish. If you are always organizing and planning and trying to keep up, when are you slowing down? Because of our busy lives and our many responsibilities and because we tend to think about the past and future a lot, our lives are limited to thinking about "real life" rather than experiencing the subtle life. If we think too much and stay too busy, we are too distracted to fully enter the subtle realm.

Our lives will consist mainly of working and thinking rather than flowing with and experiencing the love in our life.

The most powerful things that keep us from experiencing the subtle reality of love guided existence are our fast paced mentality and our habit of thinking about the past and future. The fast pace keeps us in L-mode organizing and structuring, and thoughts of past and future keep us away from being in the moment. How do we fit our spiritual insights, experiences, and desires into this type of "real life" situation? We are so caught up in L-mode thinking and busy living that when we remember or feel our spiritual essence, it seems separate from daily life. We have separated our spiritual identity from our real life identity. On some level, we know that there should only be one of us, but we stay in working, thinking L-mode for so much of the time that feeling inspired and guided and directly tied to the subtle reality of love doesn't feel like it is the real us. While we are having inspired, spiritual feelings, we know that they are real, but after the feelings leave, "real life" sets in and treats the experience like a good mood. We have thoughts like, "An inspired me is not the real me. An inspired me is just me in an inspired mood. It is true that most of the time we are separate from the subtle reality and our spiritual identity, but that does not mean that we have to be or that our spiritual identity is not the real us. The real us is our spirit inspired, slower paced, being in the moment self. We are meant to be united with our spiritual self and the subtle realm of love while we live "real life". We are just in the habit of moving too fast to stay connected to the subtle nature of reality and our spirit. Our thoughts move too quickly, our pace is too fast, and our drive to accomplish and work pushes us too hard to notice and absorb with sensitivity. We expect ourselves to feel peaceful and fulfilled in our lives, but we don't examine our approach, our thoughts, and our actions. This is the only way to make the shift to noticing the subtle.

When we look closely at L-mode thinking and realize that it drives us to act in a hurried manner, we can see that more of an R-mode approach to life will cause us to slow down. With R-mode perception, you search for depth through sensing and noticing the subtle. L-mode wants us to accomplish as much as possible, as quickly as it can. R-mode wants us to enjoy each moment and savor the experiences of life.

Before you rule out the possibility that a subtle reality or a constant connection to love and spirit are meant to exist within real life, try to imagine that possibility. Imagine living your regular life within a framework of R-mode guidelines. Imagine having some established rules that encourage you to stop thinking and planning and organizing so much. Imagine accomplishing all of your goals but at a slower, more relaxed pace. Imagine your free time being spent feeling relaxed and peaceful rather than thinking about the past and future. Imagine thinking about creative, inspirational insights rather than repeating judgmental and fearful thoughts. If you can imagine these things, I'm sure you can begin to sense how the subtle reality is where we are meant to exist. From this type of frame of mind, the beauty of life would be sensed and felt much more intensely. You would be encouraged to seek out beauty and to feel love rather than stay stuck in "real life" negative patterns of thoughts and actions. It is possible to unite with love in "real life". This is the subtle realm of existence.

When you see life through a lens of love, you know that you are going to see love in everything. The lens of love is a frame of mind.

Everyone has days where they feel on top of the world. On these days, everything looks and feels great, and when something unexpected comes up, you embrace it as an unexpected occurrence. You are surprised, alerted to, or made aware of what just happened, but you don't let the occurrence consume your attention and thinking. You are on a roll or in the flow of a great day, so you don't let yourself get caught up in negative thoughts and feelings. You remain in a strong and love filled mood. Love is always there, even if we feel compelled to judge the situation differently. If I can have a day where everything looks great and one where the same basic elements of my life make me feel overwhelmed or negative, my frame of mind or my mode of perception, not the situation, is what causes my reactions. The lens of love is a frame of mind.

If I go with the flow of the day, hold on to a love-based attitude, and try to experience each moment as it is, I will limit judgmental thoughts. When you stop trying to categorize things and accept everything as a learning experience, you free your mind from a lot of unnecessary controlling thoughts. Our role is to grow in this direction. If we continue to resist love and be fearful of life because of an overly logical and judgmental attitude, we end up trying to control too many things. Every single thing that occurs in our lives can be viewed from a logical, analytical, and judgmental frame of mind. The exact same experiences can be viewed with an open, accepting mind that stays focused on love and searching for lessons. One of the most powerful judgmental thought patterns that I have noticed about myself is my addiction to perfection. I am a very orderly and organized person, so this has really fed into my strong L-mode desire to judge my thoughts and actions. There are so many expectations that I have placed on myself because of this standard of perfection that over the years, my personal "failures" had added up to become a heavy burden. Open-mindedness! If frees you up to think in new ways. This R-mode quality helps me to continue to release the perfection baggage I've let myself carry. When I remember or discover a "less than perfect" action I've taken or quality about myself, I open my mind to loving myself as an evolving spirit. I am able to become objective about my imperfections and to forgive myself because of a love-based R-mode attitude.

When we search for the lessons in the experience, when we stay committed to feeling connected to love, when we eliminate or decrease a need to control outcomes, we are uniting ourselves with the subtle realm. The real lessons of love are learned by trying to experience love in every moment. Our frame of mind, or the way we think, affects how intensely we experience love. Every moment presents us with an opportunity to grow in our awareness of love. It may seem as though life is a series of obstacles and responsibilities, but it is meant to be more profound. The everyday reality we face can be turned around from being "real life" to being "real life" enhanced with continuous lessons of love. When you begin to change your patterns of thinking from too much L-mode to more of an R-mode approach, you loosen the grip of "real life" pain. It is possible to have entire days and even weeks where you know that you are connected to the love of the universe, and every moment is a joyous moment. When you capture this state of mind, the experiences you have seem elevated. We can let go of feeling tied down by our lives and open up to being guided. Another way to describe this elevated state or this awareness of the subtle realm is to think of it as a faith filled attitude. When your faith is strong, you know that everything will be o.k. No matter what you are facing, a painful situation or a boring or confusing time, you know that there is a purpose or a lesson in the experience. Your faith gives you certainty about where you should step next, and the uncomfortable feelings you have decrease. Faith is something we can relate to as a real experience. Most of us know what it feels like to put total trust in God or universal love. Why don't we stay in a faith filled mentality all of the time? Why do we worry and try to control outcomes rather than experience most moments with inspiration, love, and faith? We have a separation in our lives between living "real life" and being filled with faith. If we could carry our faith with us at all times, we would be seeing life through a lens of love. We would enter a whole new way of living everyday life. A subtle realm would become more obvious and real. The time we spent thinking in L-mode would lessen and open-minded, inspirational insights would replace controlling thoughts. This may sound like an unattainable goal, but discussion of this goal is a first step to making it a reality.

When we work at trying to understand that there is a subtle reality that comes through when our attitude or mode of perception is faith or love based, we open up a new world for ourselves. This new world removes us from "real life" attitudes and allows us to see life from a new perspective. The degree to which we maintain our new perspective depends on how well we understand and practice these new ways of perceiving reality. If we stay locked in a mode of being the victim of a difficult life, then that is what we will experience. We will be the victim of a difficult life. If we open up to new ways of seeing, we will experience new ways of seeing. A first step is to spend time learning about and observing our current attitudes and perceptions. Do we think and act according to L-mode type responses most of the time? If we can observe this one thing, if we can consider the possibility that we are too left brained to leave room for a right brained approach, we have revealed a powerful clue to discovering and understanding the subtle reality. We have opened up to new ways of seeing.

If my mission in life is to grow spiritually and to become more aware of how to feel and create love, I can't keep faith filled experiences separate from everyday life. I have to know that the biggest changes in my heart are going to come when I live in a moment to moment awareness of or search for the obvious and subtle qualities of love. Keeping life separate from love is something we are used to doing, but we can change this way of being. I know we can't expect ourselves to instantly know love all of the time, but we can certainly feel the presence and guidance of the universe more than we are used to feeling it now.

"Subtle reality" is a good way to describe a reality of seeing love in every moment because seeing this constant presence of love requires subtle movements and thoughts or observations. If we blaze through life with machine like qualities based in logic, speed, efficiency, and over-judgment, we miss the subtle. Subtle is slower, less obvious, and more difficult to define than our logical brains would like. The subtleties of any experience are felt more than they are expressible in words. The world is filled with subtle beauty in the form of nature. Using nature to help you become more sensitive and in tune with love and beauty is a very powerful thing to do. The more experiences you can give yourself that teach you to become absorbed in subtle beauty, the more easily you will be able to sense and enter the

subtle reality of love. When you immerse yourself in an experience with nature, you tend to want to slow down and notice
the not so obvious. The slower your pace and the more you use
R-mode, the more intensely the beauty is revealed. The word
"revealed" is important to note here because it expresses the
idea that you are not seeing the beauty because you just created it, you allowed yourself to be open to what was already
there. The beauty is revealed when we open ourselves to seeing
the beauty. We don't create the subtle beauty, we notice that it
exists. It existed before we gave it our attention, and it will exist
if we stop focusing on it. This same idea is what needs to be
applied to love. It exists always and everywhere. It has a subtle way which is powerful and beautiful, but we will not notice
the power and beauty of love unless we give it our attention.
Love will always exist. Love is a subtle part of every moment
and every experience and everything. It needs to be searched
for, and it is meant to be discovered. We need to be searching
for love for the same reasons that we need to be searching for
the subtle beauty in nature, because its subtle forms cause it
to easily go unnoticed. We tend to move too fast to notice the
subtle, and our L-mode mind keeps us thinking and acting at
that fast pace.

I can choose the degree to which I notice subtle beauty.
I can choose how much of an affect a walk in the woods will
have on me by choosing to slow down and pay attention to
the beauty. When I appreciate the depth of beauty I see, and
the fascination I feel, I am increasing my capacity to step into
the subtle realm. I am using a slower and less thought filled
R-mode frame of mind. When I draw, I look very slowly at what
I want to draw in order to shift to R-mode. I use this same skill

when I want to shift to R-mode for any reason. I pick some feeling, sound, smell, taste, touch, or visual image and try to sense and absorb its every detail. By choosing to pay attention to and appreciate the beauty in anything, I move from not noticing the subtle to becoming engaged in the moment to moment reality of the subtle realm. I have a choice about where I concentrate my attention. I may be so wound up or so used to using controlled L-mode thinking that I can't slow it down, but I have a choice to make learning this skill a priority. I can choose to spend time observing my pace, my attitudes, and my thoughts and see how and where they are guiding my attention. I can choose to notice what affects me the most and what encourages me to slow down or to speed up my thinking. I can choose to avoid people or shows or situations or conversations that carry me into habits of fast paced thinking. The goal is to become aware of what you are doing and thinking and then choose to create patterns that allow you to search for the love based subtle realm.

If I want to notice the subtle realm in "real life", I have to set this as a priority. Working at it, as a continuous practice, helps me to stay in touch with this other realm. The obvious will remain obvious, but the subtle becomes increasingly obvious when we try to give it our continuous attention. What we focus on creates our reality, so the subtle can become our reality.

Staying in touch with love requires becoming more and more aware of our perceptions of our experiences. If we examine how we perceive life or the attitude we generally carry, we will notice how often we see love as a reality and a guiding force. Having a continuous focus on searching for love means that you are staying connected to the reality of love. I can fear and try to control the unfolding of an uncontrollable situation or feel peaceful and certain that what I cannot control has a purpose. If I remain connected to love, I know I will be guided and supported towards taking the right action at the right time. When I try to control something that can't be controlled, I am working from the view that there is no larger plan. I need to stay focused on the bigger picture and ask for guidance. Instead of fighting and fearing, I need to let go to the larger force that guides us when we ask for guidance.

When you become used to letting go of things you can't control and replace the fight with requests for guidance, you step into an aspect of the subtle realm. You enter faith filled perception about your problems. This type of perception requires that you let go of your logical thought processing. When you try to let go of a frightening or confusing situation, you soon discover that it is easier said than done, but with practice and an increased awareness of R-mode you realize that faith is not logical. Faith requires trusting something abstract. Your logical mind tells you that the only way to get out of the fear, pain, and/or confusion you are facing or may be facing is to run through the situation over and over again in your mind. L-mode will take an unsolved situation and analyze it to death. It will not let go of trying to solve the problem until the problem goes away. R-mode, on the other hand, will give you the freedom to have faith over control. R-mode doesn't mind if things aren't worked out. It can imagine the bigger picture, open up to new possibilities, engage in the moment, and feel the subtleties of love and trust. R-mode allows us to trust, to imagine, and to feel the peace of love no matter what uncertainty we face. L-mode wants us to have everything worked out first. It wants us to think about how we can control the situation because it concludes that that is the only way we will be certain of the outcome. Well, all of us know that we can't control a lot of things that occur in our lives. We can enter and exist in any situation feeling fear and frustration, or we can let the situation unfold as it is meant to unfold, while maintaining faith or trusting that love will offer us support and guidance. Two different approaches can bring two very different attitudes to the exact same situation. How many times have we worried about and tried to control something beyond our control only to discover that it was happening to teach us something we really needed to know or that what we feared would happen did not occur? L-mode is responsible for our controlling types of thoughts, so becoming aware of L-mode perceptions is key to discovering the subtle realm.

The subtle realm exists on different levels. The example I just discussed shows how to enter the subtle realm through our perceptions of uncontrollable situations in our lives. The subtle realm, in this case, exists in an attitude of acceptance and faith. The subtle realm is also there on more abstract levels. When we pray or meditate in order to try to deepen our connection to our spirit, we are engaged in an exercise that gives us an opportunity to sense a higher level of love. Some exercises, such as meditation or prayer, produce more of a direct connection to the subtle realm. When the meditation is effective, you can sense love very strongly and you can have profound insights that convince you that your life and you exist within a subtle realm of love. If we carry too much thought with us during these quiet moments though, we will not be able to contact the subtle realm as intensely . as we may wish. L-mode must be released. Let's go back to one of the drawing exercises for a moment. When I explained the pure contour drawing exercise, I was giving an example of the most intense or highest level of R-mode experience you could have while drawing. Pure contour drawing carries you almost completely away from L-mode because you draw very detailed lines at an extremely slow pace. Since you never take your eyes off the subject you are drawing, your L-mode doesn't have a chance to pop up and criticize what you have drawn. Instead of focusing on the outcome or what you are creating, your attention remains absolutely fixed on seeing finer and more subtle details in the lines you are observing. This same R-mode intensity applies during prayer, quiet time, nature experiences, or meditation. These are exercises that give you the opportunity to almost completely quiet L-mode thinking by allowing yourself to focus totally on the subtle. When meditating, you are not trying to do anything except focus totally on a subtle feeling of love. You have the opportunity to turn off L-mode and experience the more elevated emotions, sensations, and insights of love. You have slowed down and have become quiet and able to concentrate all of your attention on experiencing the subtle reality of love. The intensity of this experience is directly tied to your ability to quiet your L-mode thinking, and it is one of the most effective exercises there is for making a connection to a higher level of the subtle realm. The key to having success with these meditation exercises is to remain absolutely fixed on the FEELINGS of love in your heart. When you feel love by imaging that you can trust, and are supported and guided by love, you remove the L-mode THOUGHTS of whether or not you can trust or feel love. When you imagine the love, you enter the feeling of it, and you begin to exist in the subtle realm. This is "being". Feeling love, this real feeling, is being in love or "being". We enter the subtle realm when we are "being".

I realize that we spend most of our time consumed by daily activities and thoughts that are removed from the subtle realm experience of meditation and prayer, but the love we feel during our meditations and/or prayers will carry over into our daily life activities and remind us to search for the love-based subtle realm. The subtle realm of love always exists. We need to continue to draw our attention towards it on as many levels as we can so that we can maintain a frame of mind or mode of perceiving reality that constantly includes an awareness of love. Our goal should be to have our obvious reality become immersed in the subtle reality of love. When we search for the existence of love in every experience, we open ourselves to seeing each of those experiences as being part of a spiritual journey.

CHAPTER 6

Negative Influences

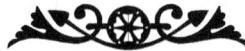

A nything that removes you from searching for and feeling love should be examined. There are many influences common to most people that remove us from love. Some of these influences are more obvious than others. Some of the more obvious examples of thoughts and experiences that have the potential to discourage us from perceiving love have to do with money, negative images and words, fear of death, a lack of guidelines about moral judgment, and misplaced priorities. When we examine our lives, we see that what we think about and how we think is strongly influenced by things outside of ourselves. We need to pay close attention to whom or what we are influenced by before we can take charge of our lives. What we consider to be helpful or harmful must be identified, and then we can try to prevent ourselves from being too influenced by harmful experiences.

Years ago, I decided to stop reading newspapers and watching certain television shows. This was difficult to do at first because I had bought into the notion that being uninformed about most news events meant that you lacked a certain intelligence. This sounds so ridiculous to me now, but I actually had to convince myself that it was o.k. to be uninformed about news events. I didn't have to be embarrassed about not knowing this information. The reason I removed television news and newspapers from my life is because they often had such a negative impact on my emotions and thoughts. They pulled me away from trusting and feeling love. I still avoid newspapers completely and 90% of television news because it takes too much energy to keep them from negatively influencing my thoughts and emotions.

A negative influence removes your faith and trust in the guidance of love. If you base decisions on negative influences, you will take actions that lead your life off the universally designed path. We should be trying to stay on a path which is guided by our sense of right action. A right action gives you a gut level feeling that resonates with love, so avoiding influences that remove you from feeling and trusting love makes right action much more possible. Obviously, we can't be constantly pondering every action or thought we engage in, but we can look at some of the larger or more highly impacting influences in our lives with regard to whether or not they are a negative influence.

The first question we should ask ourselves is "What are my goals?". Then we should set our priorities in accordance with these goals. I am assuming that each of us wants the same life goal of becoming more spiritually evolved. This is a goal we may not verbalize too often, but no matter where we are or what we have accomplished, the most important mission we are faced with is to unravel the mysteries of our spiritual essence. We know this at a soul level. So, if spiritual awareness is our main purpose in life, it has to be our guide for all of our other priorities. This does not mean that we have to speak of it constantly, it just has to create the foundation for all of our other priorities and goals.

The list of priorities most of us have is inspired by our basic needs. We need to physically and emotionally survive, and we have to play a role in caring for others and the earth. Money plays a big part in our need for survival, but money can take over our lives and push spiritual growth aside. When thoughts and actions that are tied to money cause us to forget our spiritual essence, money becomes a negative influence. It is so easy to get caught up in money related issues because the logic and pace of L-mode keep us convinced that our physical existence is our only reality and therefore our greatest priority. Also, it is easy to be distracted by money because we need to pay bills, buy groceries, buy clothes, pay for school and work related costs, health care, and many more basic survival expenses. We are forced to think about money every day. It is the most all pervading necessity in our lives. Of course we will tend to be somewhat awed by and fearful of money because of the power it has to affect our lives. But, if our awe or fears of money become too great, our thoughts and actions will become negative. Money becomes a negative influence in our lives when we allow ourselves to be overly influenced by its power. Money is powerful, but it does not have to overpower our thoughts and actions. We can choose to limit the influence money has over our thoughts and actions. We can keep money as a priority and not let it become a negative influence. The thing to remember is that spiritual evolution is our main priority. It comes before everything else in our lives. Since we need money, we have to learn how to limit its negative influence over us in order to leave room for spiritual awareness. The way to do this is to remember that we have to keep things in perspective. We need to remind ourselves that money is a necessity, but it does not define us, and it is not our biggest power. Our biggest power is accessed when we connect to love and spiritual guidance. Money is a means of survival, but it is not what gives us our direction or sense or right action. Right action comes through when we are connected to love, and right action empowers us by connecting us to universal power. Universal power is our biggest power. When we follow right action or love motivated action, we are tapping into the limitless power of the universe. I am still trying to let go of my fear of money. It has had such power over me for so long that it has often prevented me from trusting love and the guidance and power of the universe. I'm sure that most of my fears about money reached their greatest depths while I was a young adult. Being a single mother at such a young age created many financial hardships that my son and I had to endure. My fears about survival and providing for my son were so enormous that I was often in a state of panic. I was overwhelmed by my responsibilities and didn't have the emotional and spiritual maturity to be able to cope with my situation. Since these patterns were so deeply set, I am still working on releasing my fears about money. Certainly, most people fear the power money has to control their standard of life, but when you have experienced extreme financial hardships for many years, you will likely have developed a deep fear of money. Now that I have trained myself to trust the universe, my negative responses to money related difficulties have become less frequent. I still become overwhelmed by my financial pressures some times, but now I know what to do when these negative thoughts take over my mind. I know, at those times, that I have to trust and feel love. I get back on track by slowing down and forcing myself to feel the presence of peace in my heart. Sometimes, I have to imagine that I feel love before I can actually feel it, and then, after a while, I begin to remember how to trust love and release fear.

Another money related issue we should watch for is how it can drive us to work at too fast or intense a pace. If we work in moderation in order to slow down our pace and stay with a program of spiritually rooted practices, we strengthen our feelings of connection to a universal plan and feel guided and more fulfilled and complete than we would if we didn't do those things. If we are leading an existence that doesn't require that we work for or worry about money, we can choose to be obsessed with possessions and things and to give them our constant attention and thoughts, or we can give spiritual growth its place as a priority in our life. A person with a lot of money runs the risk of forgetting their spiritual essence because they can end up thinking of their material possessions and powers more than their power of spirit. Their lives are filled with opportunities for pleasurable experiences, so their need to seek the love of spirit is not so obvious to them. If they begin to feel empty or lonely and unhappy, even with all of their money and possessions, they may begin to notice that there is a power or force larger than money. Although money is extremely powerful, there is no way that it can complete us spiritually. The universal plan and the underlying unity of life runs on love not money.

These ideas show that money has great power to influence what we focus on and how we think and feel. The ideas also point out that the power of money cannot compare to the power of spirit. When we choose to place spiritual evolution as a priority over money, we are choosing to keep the negative power of money from blinding us from the power of spirit. Money can easily become a negative influence in our lives because of its power and our dependence on it for survival. Keeping our dependency and need for money in perspective by not letting it control us with fears and misplaced priorities is a healthier way to approach life.

Another potentially negative influence is too much negative information. We get a lot of our information from newspapers, radio, and television. The medium that influences us most directly is television. This is a high impact medium because it gives us words and pictures. For the most part, the shows and articles that have the greatest potential for carrying negative information are news based shows. We are given daily doses of powerful information about disasters and crimes. This is, for the most part, what has come to be defined as news. News is generally an unveiling of stories about human, economic, and environmental tragedies. We don't need to be reminded, almost hourly, of negative images and situations, but we continue to support this type of broadcasting by watching these shows. We have become so accustomed to seeing tragedy that we accept it as part of our daily diet of information. How many of us take the time to consider the impact negative news has on our patterns of thinking? For example, if we have been watching an hour of negative news, do we think about whether this will affect the thoughts we will have and the actions we will take after we've finished watching the show? If I look at tragedies too often without first preparing myself, I will become influenced by a negative way of perceiving. As I have already mentioned, I avoid negative news as much as possible. I am concerned with what is going on in the world, but I have to draw the line at some point. With all of the particulars of my life and the lives of my family and friends, I need to be very careful about where I put my attention and energy. We have to be careful about the images and words we allow into our mind. Letting ourselves follow stories of control, deception, injustice, and tragedies that cause undeserved pain to others can encourage fear based and hopeless thoughts. If these same stories were given to us with helpful guidelines about how to put them into a love-based perspective, they wouldn't have as much potential to become a negative influence. When you see only the hopeless side of a tragedy, you need to feed yourself the necessary thoughts to turn the tragedy into a lesson of love. You need to see the bigger picture, and this takes time and energy. The only way I can keep a relaxed and inspired pace in my life and mind and still meet my responsibilities is by conserving my energy and using it wisely. I have to decide what is most deserving of my attention so that I don't feel as though I'm usually running on empty. Seeing only the tragedy and not feeding yourself love based, universal purpose thoughts puts you in a more likely position to be negatively influenced. The number of negative stories in an average news broadcast is far greater than the number of stories about acceptance and love. Murders, trials, wars, illnesses, wrongdoings, tragedies, and disasters of the world are occurring all of the time, but thinking about them every day really pulls us away from developing a less fearful mind. If you are trying to teach yourself how to have an "in the moment" awareness of the beauty of life, you are putting unnecessary obstacles in your way by having daily doses of negative news.

If a viewer is presented with a television show that encourages them to relax and to slow down the pace of their mind and life, to have an expanded more open-minded attitude, or to let go of trying to control outcomes in order to be open to a feeling of being guided, then they could learn positive lessons from these R-mode experiences and then apply them to their own life. When a show is filled with overly judgmental, controlling, fast paced, and/or overly analytical L-mode thoughts and ways, the viewer is subjecting themselves to unnecessary negativity. The reason I am mentioning this is because there are so many different television shows that display these L-mode patterns. Television has the power to intensify and increase negative L-mode thought patterns, and most people don't know enough about L-mode to consider this fact. When L-mode is presented with something, it breaks it down, analyzes it, judges it, and places it into a category. It looks at situations as facts, information, and images and not as an opportunity to search for the subtle details and beauty. Since we are using L-mode most of the time, we have to assume that when we watch television and see something negative, we will analyze, judge, categorize, and logically think through what we have seen. In most cases, this is too much time spent thinking about something negative. L-mode loves to be busy, so the more information we feed ourselves, the harder it works. If the information is depressing or negative, L-mode will still keep working. Why don't we limit the amount of negative information we give ourselves in order to decrease our number of negative thoughts? When we learn how to use R-mode, we will be drawn towards positive responses when faced with negative information. R-mode will help us to slow down and become aware of our more subtle and elevated emotions and thoughts.

One potentially negative subject or influence that does come up very frequently on television and in movies is death.

Most of the time, these presentations of death are not positive. Do we realize how often we are exposing ourselves to death as a negative concept? Not only do we expose ourselves to negative images of death, but also, we rarely have discussions about the reality of death. Our lives need to include respect for and education about death because death is a part of our reality. We discuss disease and illness, but we rarely discuss the reality of death. I'm sure part of this avoidance comes from our fear of dying, but when we allow ourselves to see negative images of death, these images are increasing our fear of death. If we want to learn to accept death, we need to examine the death images we see and ask ourselves if they are healthy images. Do we benefit from seeing them, or should we try to avoid these images? Also, we need to discuss our mortality.

My attitude towards death has changed dramatically over the years. I used to think that death was unfair. I was in my early 20's when my grandmother on my mother's side died. The thing that stands out most in my mind about her death was my refusal to accept the justice of her death. When I attended her wake, I refused to look at her remains because they represented that injustice. Her remains were not her. She had been pulled away, and we were expected to accept this lifeless body as her replacement. To me, this was not fair. I couldn't even vaguely imagine where she had gone. Her leaving was so difficult for me to understand in a logical way that it seemed like she really wasn't gone. She had just gone missing. It sort of felt like she had been taken away and was being held captive at some other place. As far as I was concerned, her disappearance was completely incomprehensible and therefore unjust. Her death affected me more deeply than any other death I've experienced, but all of them struck me as being unreal and unfair. As my understanding of my spiritual nature grew, I began to feel peace at greater depths. Love began to reveal itself as a state of mind, and I learned that this state carried me into another realm or way of perceiving. I used this state to understand illogical issues like death, and it was at this point that I was able to release my confusion and anger towards it. I am no longer confused about where we go once we pass on. I think of it as a transition to another realm where love and wisdom are always present. Someone I care for may leave me physically, and I will have to suffer through the pain of that loss, but I have felt connected to universal love enough to feel at home with it and to be happy for those who have fully entered in to that realm. I embrace death now because I know that it is orchestrated by the love of the universe.

We have to remember that our logical mind has control of our perceptions most of the time. If we see negative images of death, our logic tells us that death is negative. Also, since L-mode logic sees this life as the only reality in existence, it does not make sense to consider that we can, after death, enter a realm where we will still exist. My logical thinking tells me that if I can't know what it will be like when I die, then nothing exists after death. R-mode will give us an opportunity to imagine another realm beyond this one, and love can carry us to that other way of knowing. If we can imagine that we are love, then we can imagine that we will exist in love after we die. Logic tells us that any existence after death is impossible, but when we learn to trust love, we realize that love is what created us and that it will always exist. We will realize that we are functioning on a physical level with rules of logic guiding most of our perceptions but that love can fit into this logic. Love is the ever-lasting force that allowed us to be born and to live the here and now, and it is what will carry us beyond this physical existence.

It takes an open mind to consider and understand these ideas. They don't make sense logically until you experience them. With the help of R-mode perception, you can suspend logic and doubt and experience love as your true nature. When you experience even a small piece of your true nature, the force of universal love, you can carry the memory of this experience with you into your daily life and use it to try to convince L-mode that love exists after death.

The more R-mode experiences we have that allow us to turn off the logic and analysis of our L-mode thinking and the more experiences we have of connecting to love, the greater our chances are of accepting death. We have to recognize that death is extremely difficulty to understand, let alone accept, if we are looking at it from a purely logical perspective. Our connections with the subtle realm or universal love can reveal death to be a transition point, not an end to life.

The death and violence we are exposed to on television and in movies is not encouraging us to try to understand the true nature of death. The images we see are usually violent. This encourages viewers to have an irreverence for life and to fear death. When you see someone being shot or murdered in a casual yet violent way, do you feel fear and discomfort or love and reverence for life and death? It is instinctive for us to feel fear when faced with violence. Also, when life and death are not treated with love and respect, death seems unjust. We have to be careful about encouraging the idea that death is unfair if we want to learn to understand and accept death as a natural, spiritual progression. We should try to approach death with an open mind and a loving heart. Anything that discourages this type of approach is a negative influence. When you consider the importance of learning to understand and accept death, you realize that any image of death should be taken seriously. Death becomes a negative influence when it is removed from love.

Moral judgment can also become a negative influence. It can cause us to miss out on the loving acceptance of ourselves and others. Morals are standards of conduct we consider to be right. We consider them to something we can use to help ourselves evolve spiritually. If we were raised to follow moral standards of conduct, we find ourselves in situations every day where we feel we have to judge if something is right or wrong. If we want to progress spiritually, we have to use judgment and our intuition to guide our behavior, but too much judgment can make it difficult to accept and forgive. Moral standards are necessary, but they can become a negative influence if we base them on overly judgmental views of right and wrong.

Our tendency is to see things as black and white. We like to categorize things, and the less complex the categories, the easier it is to keep track of everything. This is, of course, an L-mode characteristic. As predominantly L-mode driven creatures, we love to judge and organize things into neat and easy to label categories. Right and wrong are so cut and dry that L-mode loves this way of viewing things. When we come across some situation we believe we must judge, we have to be very cautious about whether or not we are being too quick to assess and categorize with a black and white mentality. Right and wrong or black and white don't leave room for grey areas. Most things in life have many components or factors that should be considered. Just because we tend to want to place things into two general groups does not mean that this is the only way or the healthiest way to judge. When we approach any issue or ourselves or others with morally based questions, love has to precede judgment. If we look at everything in search of its essential nature of love first and follow our intuition, we will have guarded against being overly judgmental. Not only do we decrease the likelihood of us being too judgmental, we increase the chances that we will be able to see more clearly and deeply in to the situation.

Before I understood the power of my L-mode mind, I was totally unaware of how possible it is to forgive myself. I had been very hard on myself. I judged things I did with a strict right/wrong mentality. Essentially, what I was doing was not loving myself. If this was the standard I was setting for myself, then certainly I was using this standard on others. After realizing that this method of over judgment was coming from L-mode, I was able to detach myself from its powerful grasp. My response to my self-criticism had been to think of it as a personality trait. I just happened to be that type of person. It was such a relief for me to understand that that was not the case. I could choose to turn off L-mode. "It" or "its" method did not define me as a person. I am beyond, or more powerful than, the responses and conclusions made by my overly judgmental mind. It was a gradual process, but eventually I was able to love myself. The anger and guilt I had felt towards myself decreased so much that I was shocked. I couldn't believe that I had allowed myself to put up with so much pain. Once you understand the qualities of L-mode, you realize that learning to love and forgive ourselves can be much easier than it seems. Knowing this brings me tremendous relief. I can judge my thoughts and actions with an open mind and a loving heart. I am actually allowed to be accepting of every single thing about myself. I look at changes I need to make as growth exercises and have stopped expecting myself to be flawless. When I see myself this way, I am learning to have this view towards every single action of every single person in existence. Moral judgment takes on a new meaning when you look at it this way. We are not the judge and jury of everyone else's life. We are choice makers that have to choose love first and then wait to be guided to our next thought or action. We can choose to judge others and ourselves as being right or wrong, or we can choose to first feel love and compassion. The reason I am focusing on this is because overly judgmental behavior is at the root of so many shows and topics of conversation. If we look closely at a lot of what we see, I'm sure we will conclude that judgment is being over used. We shouldn't feel badly about our tendency to judge too quickly or to over judge. Instead, we can see it as having an over active L-mode. An overly judgmental mind needs to be treated with R-mode awareness, not self-reprimand and more overly judgmental thoughts. Take a step back when you are judging yourself or others too quickly or too harshly, and try to become more relaxed and open-minded. Your priority is to turn down L-mode and turn up R-mode. Try to search for love first, and this will open your mind to seeing in new ways. Moral issues can be argued based on differences in our backgrounds, and people should be held accountable for non-loving, immoral acts. We just have to remember that we are always supposed to love, no matter what. If our thoughts or actions don't leave room for love and forgiveness, we are staying stuck. If we want to move forward in our spiritual evolution, then we move nearer to love. Our capacity to label things as right and wrong and to judge quickly is so intense because of our dominant L-mode. Our R-mode capacity to be open-minded and to imagine will help us increase our thoughts of loving forgiveness and acceptance. Moral awareness is an essential part of our spiritual evolution, but it becomes a negative influence or hindrance to our growth if we judge before we love. When you place love in front of judgment, and ask for guidance from the universe, the choices you must make become clear.

We need to pay close attention to whom or what we are influenced by before we can take charge of our lives. Negative influences can be very powerful, especially ones relating to money, negative information, death, over judgment, and misplaced priorities. Our response to negative influences should always be that love comes first.

CHAPTER 7

Loneliness and Being Alone

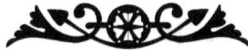

Everyone knows what loneliness feels like. It can arise when you lose someone to death or after a significant relationship has ended or been temporarily disconnected in some fashion. We can miss having a mate relationship or having close relationships with friends and family members. These are painful and real situations that do generate feeling of loneliness. We need and will long for love from others. The loneliness I want to discuss is deeper than these examples. It is something we rarely discuss because it is difficult to recognize and even harder to face. I label it fundamental loneliness. I had no idea about this deep form of loneliness until I went through a period in my life where I almost completely isolated myself from other people. This period occurred shortly after my divorce. I felt vulnerable and wanted to protect myself, and I was very busy at home with two small children and a teenager. I knew that I had to be very careful about where I put my energy. For a period of about two and one half years, I intentionally cut myself off from some people and really limited my interaction with almost everyone else, including my family and close friends. I didn't look for or even consider having a mate relationship. I created

99

this protected living environment because I believed I had to do this. (I am definitely not trying to promote extreme isolation experiences. My personal needs and desires led me to do this.) At first, my pains of loneliness were tied to missing adult relationships, but, as time went by, this changed. My loneliness began to be directed towards me. I missed myself! I realized that I longed for a more real and heart-felt connection to my spirit. I was shocked by how lonely I felt. I had been covering up the tremendous depth of this feeling for a long time. It was a painful and overwhelming feeling, but I faced it because I knew that dealing with this was a very important part of my spiritual growth. The more I faced this feeling, the more I realized that it came out of a need to feel more closely identified with my spirit. Although I had been the type of person who liked spending time alone, and I did practice meditation exercises, I hadn't been making a strong enough connection with my spirit. I had often gone through very uncomfortable meditation sessions but had never understood why the emotional discomfort arose. If I became too uncomfortable, I would distract myself with some other activity. Now I was finally able to label and face the pain. I was lonely at a fundamental level. I had to learn to identify more closely with my spirit and make it more personal and real. During this period of time, I gradually learned how to meditate more effectively. I learned that I had to focus on feelings of love in my heart and then think of that love as being my true identity or spirit. This helped make my spirit seem real. The more often and deeply I made this connection, the less lonely I felt. I began to realize that the pain I had felt from missing my spirit had been so intense that I had never let myself feel it completely. Subconsciously, I had blocked out the depth of my loneliness. It is very likely that most of us are suffering from this fundamental loneliness unless we have made a conscious effort to regularly and directly feel love as our identity. Our spirit needs to become real to us, or we will suffer. Also, I have come to understand that when we forget or never learn to identify closely with our spirit, we can sense a void or have an awareness that something is missing. We will be confused by and driven to fill this void.

When we are alone and undistracted, fundamental loneliness will begin to surface. Because of the intensity of this feeling, many people avoid being alone. How many of us are comfortable being alone for any significant period of time? We don't want to spend too much time alone because we don't want to feel lonely. Whether it is subconscious or conscious, our habit of avoiding this feeling is directly tied to how busy we become, the relationships we choose, the material "things" we desire, etc.. We are trying to avoid pain and fill a void if we have not made a strong connection to our spirit. Fundamental loneliness needs to be addressed because it can affect our daily thoughts and actions and therefore the path of our spiritual evolution.

Everything we experience and perceive in our lives is colored by how closely we are connected to our spirit. If we know how to connect to our spirit, we can make sure that our decisions are based on healthy choices rather than a desire to escape our fundamental feelings of loneliness. If, for example, we know that we still feel a void in our heart and know that we need to further connect to our own spirit, we won't rush into mate relationships. We recognize that loneliness is first to be addressed from a position of loving ourselves. After we know how to better connect to our spirit, our fundamental lonely feelings will decrease, and we will be drawn to relationships because of healthy feelings and reasons. Another way that fundamental loneliness can appear in our daily lives is through our money and activity choices. These choices may be coming from a desire to fill a void. If we are aware of the idea that we may have a void within us that comes from a lack of connection to our spirit, we know that a feeling of emptiness like this cannot be filled with activities or things we buy. When we feel a need to buy or do something in order to make ourselves feel better, we could examine those needs more closely and, if necessary, look for ways to feel connected to our spirit.

Probably the most difficult thing to remember when you feel a void or deep loneliness is that you won't feel whole unless you connect to your spirit. We are so trained to look outside of ourselves when we feel lonely or empty that it seems illogical to search within. L-mode wants us to be logical, and it bases its logic on stored information and logical equations. If we define loneliness as a terrible feeling we get when we are alone, logic dictates that we remove loneliness by not being alone. Logic dictates that we fill a void with things that make us feel good. What is missing from these logical formulas is the fact that we have separated ourselves from our true identity when we feel a void or when fundamental loneliness overcomes us, and someone or something cannot replace making that connection to our essential nature. When we learn and accept that this does make sense, we can more easily turn to ourselves when we suffer from fundamental loneliness.

In order to turn back to yourself and feel more connected to your spirit, you need to quiet your mind and still yourself so that you are not distracted. Most of the time it is difficult to stop the mind, specifically L-mode, from thinking, but this is the only way we can make a strong connection to our spirit. If we realize that we need to connect to our spirit, and we quiet ourselves and our surroundings, the next step is to be willing to confront the pain and fight off the fears and anxiety of facing our loneliness. L-mode hates it when we are still, and it wants us to solve problems with analysis and logic. If we decide to sit still and face our lonely feelings, L-mode will still want to be in charge and will encourage us to analyze what we are feeling and why we feel such pain. Instead of thinking about how and why loneliness exists, move straight to focusing on love. If we get into the pain we have in our heart from feeling a void for too long, we can get stuck there in justifying and trying to figure out the pain. Turn to an R-mode state of mind, and open up to experiencing love in the moment. Concentrate on feeling love in your heart, and wait for yourself to absorb deeper and deeper emotional connections to love and then imagine that you are making a connection to your spirit. If we don't take the time to recognize that loneliness has to be dealt with by direct connection to love, our spiritual essence, we will put the pain and symptoms of loneliness in a position where they may become more powerful.

Being alone is something most of us tend to avoid. How often do we spend several hours alone, in silence, without other people? Most likely there is a fear of facing deep lonely feelings, and this drives us to stay busy and to avoid being alone. Also, because the pace of life that we have created is so fast, we believe that we don't have time to spend "doing nothing", but is that how we should be viewing time alone? Should we place time alone near the top or bottom of our list of priorities? How can we expect ourselves to be guiding our lives by spiritually grounded choices if we don't maintain a regular and close connection to our spirit? We need to remember that we are here for a reason and that we are supported and guided by the love of the universe. How can we maintain this faith and believe that our spirit is real unless we spend time alone on a regular basis trying to make that connection? If I think that I am too busy to try to make a strong connection to my spirit every day, I tell myself that I should examine my priorities and that I'm sure I can shift things around to give myself some time every day to meditate. If we do this every day, we will begin to define and relate to our spirit in a more concrete way.

It took my experience of isolation for me to discover how much I missed myself, my real spiritual self. Now that I know this, I look forward to spending as much time alone as I can. Unless I'm in a really stressed mood, I can pretty well always remember how necessary it is to sit alone and feel a strong connection to my spirit. As I have said, I am the type of person who enjoys solitude, but I use those experiences in a different way now. I used to love to sit alone just to relax my mind and body. I loved "taking in" nature experiences. I still do these things, but now, my first interest is to focus as intensely as I can on feeling love. Then I try to feel as though that place of love is my identity, my home. My aim is to really believe that love is where I come from, and it is the core of my identity. WE ARE LOVE. It requires concentration to keep those feeling and thoughts sustained, but I have found that gradually my spirit has become more concrete and less abstract. My spirit is no longer just a thought. It has become as solid and real as the love in my heart.

We are a society that moves at a fast pace. People rarely slow down, and our society sends out the message that if we are not busy, we are wasting time. (L-mode promotes this type of thinking.) But, being busy and forcing ourselves to keep up with everything encourages us to ignore our loneliness. Logically, it makes sense that the harder we work the more we accomplish, but what are we working towards? What are our goals? Do we want controlled and orderly perfection in our work and home environment, or do we want to learn how to connect to our spirit and let it guide our actions? We are a "take charge" type of society. If something isn't working or something is lacking in our lives, we are taught to make it happen through determination and hard work. Of course we need to be self-disciplined and to work consistently at accomplishing tasks and goals, but being reflective and quiet is equally important. In school, at work, and in our homes, we are not training ourselves to stay in touch with our spirit. We are so convinced that we control our destiny by working hard, we don't even talk about how valuable "quiet alone time" can be. How can we expect ourselves to recognize loneliness for what it is, our spirit crying for our attention, if we are too busy? How can we expect ourselves to be making decisions that fall in line with our best interests if we are not regularly relating to and consulting our spirit? L-mode pushes us to think and act in overly fast and controlling ways. When we learn that L-mode does not have to be our dictator, we can keep ourselves from staying too busy. If we begin to approach each day as a journey rather than a series of tasks that have to be completed, we will open our minds to seeing our lives differently. We are meant to be spiritually driven, not task driven. When we identify mainly with our busy, working mode, we can't develop a strong connection to our spiritual identity.

Take some time to sit back and relax. Try to relax enough so that you can concentrate on having a neutral examination of yourself. Maybe you will discover that you have been spending too much time trying to be perfect with your daily accomplishments. Maybe you will realize that you have been working too hard, so hard that you never spend time alone. If you avoid being alone, try to examine what you fear about being alone. Maybe you are afraid of your loneliness. After some reflection, you may realize that no matter how many goals you set and accomplish, you still don't feel satisfied. There are so many ways we busy ourselves, and we have so many responsibilities and high standards set for ourselves, that all of us need to sit back and reflect on these issues.

L-mode convinces us that control, perfection, and order are the only ways of filling the void and moving forward. If you let go of that idea and reduce L-mode's hold over you, you are left with an opportunity to deal with what is actually missing, a personal connection to your spirit. R-mode will help us make that connection because it lets us sit still and perceive things in new ways. If we are afraid to sit alone because we fear our thoughts or feelings, we can use an R-mode activity to turn our attention towards feeling love. When you choose to be quiet, put some beautiful music on or sit outside in a natural setting. You could even look out the window and watch the clouds drift by. The main thing you want to accomplish is a connection to love. After you feel love, you practice thinking of this love as your spirit and true identity. You can look at or listen to or imagine anything beautiful and connect to this beauty by feeling love. The stronger and more often you feel the love, the more closely you will be able to identify with your spirit. It's easy to do this if you are used to turning off L-mode, but most of us have too many L-mode thoughts that stay with us even when we try to focus on loving feelings. L-mode makes us think too much and R-mode encourages us to feel the moment. Practicing making the shift to R-mode in as many situations as possible will teach you how to let go of L-mode. Using nature as a tool can really help us make the shift to R-mode. All that is natural has an energy or beauty radiating from it, and we can connect to this peaceful, inspiring energy by searching for it and respecting it. Really looking for the beauty or energy and wanting to connect to it turns off L-mode. The energy is often so subtle that our fast paced L-mode can't sense it. L-mode does not like to slow down, so if we calmly and slowly look for beauty in the subtle details of nature, L-mode will eventually let go and R-mode will take over. Once you sense the beauty of nature, you increase your connection to it through further and further recognition and appreciation of this beauty. Nature has such powerful beauty, and we are structured to feel very close to or part of this. It is something that captures our heart. It fills all of our senses to a point where we can connect to it in a very complete way. We can sense the beauty with our eyes, with our ears, with our nose, etc. The beauty or pure energy of nature is brought to us through our senses. When we fill up with the beauty of nature, we are filling up with love. The emotional contentment and euphoric feelings we get from appreciating something pure and beautiful is an expression or form of love. Nature provides us with helpful and powerful opportunities to turn off unwanted L-mode thoughts and to move directly to love and our spiritual identity.

So much of our spiritual growth is based on how well we understand and take charge of ourselves. Are we going to let life push us along, or are we going to realize that we can choose how we approach life? Avoiding fundamental loneliness is a powerful example of how life can push us along. I can choose to be aware of this and be watchful for ways that I may be trying to avoid the pain of this loneliness. Am I running from spending time alone, am I trying to fill a void, or am I listening to the voice of my spirit when it calls to me through lonely feelings? It is definitely an ongoing process for me, but knowing what I should watch for is extremely helpful.

Being alone is sometimes very difficult for me. When I notice this happening, it sends off warning bells. I am alerted to the fact that it may be very possible that I need to be alone. I have probably been working too hard and have been ignoring a soul felt relationship with myself. L-mode can put us on automatic pilot so easily that often we slip into a busy mode without being aware of it and stay there for too long. Not only do we have to cherish our time alone, but we have to be on guard against having too much of the fast pace and busy thoughts of L-mode.

Once we know that we have to watch for and pay attention to signs of fundamental loneliness, we have taken a giant step forward in our advancement towards spiritual awareness. Loneliness is rarely discussed in this context, but it is one the most important things we can understand about our spirit. Not only are we supposed to have respect for and pay attention to loneliness, we need to search for ways in which we tend to avoid it or mask its presence. If we are bored, hate being alone, are always trying to stay busy, are buying things just to make ourselves feel better, keep waiting for fulfillment to arrive, have a void we can't describe or fill, or think others are to blame for the fact that we don't feel complete and totally loved, etc., we need to discover more about fundamental loneliness. Our relationships, our work, and our responsibilities have to be put on hold for a period of time each day so that we can remember our essence. Between L-mode pace, control, and logic and our determination to fill an internal void and to avoid being alone and feeling our fundamental loneliness, we are driving ourselves further and further away from understanding and facing the message loneliness is trying to teach. Loneliness brings the message that WE NEED TO FOCUS ON OUR SPIRIT. We need to be driven by our spirit, not L-mode, and we do this by identifying more closely with love.

We make our spirit more real when we meditate on love and try to think of this as our identity; therefore, we should have a period of time each day where we meditate on feeling connected to love, but we also need to connect to love in more casual ways. For example, we can begin to notice how we are perceiving something and figure out if we should have a more expanded or open-minded approach that reminds us of our spirit. We can examine our pace. Is L-mode driving us to move too fast, and is this keeping us out of touch with our spirit? If we are rushing around the house or office thinking about all of the things we still have to accomplish during the rest of the day, we could change our thoughts and think that maybe we will move at a pace that feels less hurried in order to keep our attention in the moment. If we stop thinking so much about what else has to be done, we can remember that we have people and experiences right in front of us that can be loved. We can search for the joy in the moment and give our L-mode planning a rest. This is a more casual way of connecting to our spirit than meditation, but it is very effective. When we search for the love in any moment and begin feeling it, we are strengthening our connection to our spirit. Another way we could connect to love is by noticing if we are continuously repeating thoughts of anger or frustration about things we can't control, and then we can choose to try and decrease them. If something I cannot control is causing me to get locked into an angry or frustrated mood, I am distancing myself from my spirit. Choosing to let go of what we can't control pulls us towards our spirit. I know that it is very difficult to keep from feeling frustrated about things we desperately want to control, but understanding and using R-mode techniques helps us connect to peace and love. R-mode can be used to help us see a situation in a new way or to understand reasons why things happen. It is willing to suspend logic and go with intuition. It helps us slow down and become absorbed in feeling subtle feelings of love and peace and to have thoughts of inspiration.

We can remember and get to know our spirit during our regular daily life experiences by feeling love and by doing loving and healthy things for ourselves and others. As I have mentioned, we can also use meditation for a more direct method of connecting to our spirit. Meditation gives us the opportunity to clearly recognize and directly face fundamental loneliness and then to move towards developing a more concrete relationship with and definition of our spirit.

My spiritual identity has become the love I feel. It is very concrete because I feel it as a real sensation in my heart and an inner knowing of rightness or instincts. Now, I carry a greater confidence about the path I am on because I feel guided by something real. My spirit is not an abstract idea. Because my spirit is now part of me rather than something vague and removed from me, I have a greater sense that I am part of the universal system of love. I have the power of this love to help me through my life, and I know that I am not alone. I don't always act and think in this way, but I remember and identify with my spirit and universal love more frequently and with greater intensity than I ever have before. Becoming aware of my fundamental loneliness played a key role in helping me learn to identify more closely with my spirit.

CHAPTER 8

Our True Selves

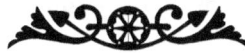

Who am I? This is a very important question. How many of us ask ourselves this question? If we examine ourselves very closely, we realize that we change our definition of who we are, to some degree, as the years progress. Also, we grow in our awareness of ourselves over the years, and this self understanding shapes what we consider to be our identity. But, most of us have not been taught that our spirit is our true identity. We are more than our personality.

All people come from the same source and will return to that source once they die. The quest of life is to educate ourselves in ways that teach us to remember our source while we are alive on earth. Spiritual development requires that we mold and shape our individual selves into spiritually aware beings. We do this by becoming more aware of our source and by learning to make it an integral part of our identity. Our true self includes our personality and our spiritual source. We are unique individuals with individual quirks, characteristics, and needs, and purposes but we are more importantly part of the loving energy of the universe.

Usually, we associate ourselves with our individual self and not so much with our universal self. The source of everything in existence is the energy of love, so we should include this essential or true nature as a fundamental part of our identity. We are made of the energy of the universe, and we can feel or experience our true self by feeling and experiencing love. It sounds so simple, and it is that simple. The goal in spiritual evolution is to know and experience love so much that you begin to feel that you are love. You identify so closely with love that love becomes the foundation of your identity. The same source that created you still remains as your essential nature. Forgetting this pulls you away from love and remembering this helps you to evolve towards becoming more of your true self.

If these concepts sound too abstract, remember that L-mode cannot absorb illogical concepts. When we try to present ourselves with abstract concepts, we need to resist the temptation to criticize or reject them based on the fact that they seem abstract and/or illogical. L-mode constantly reminds us that we have to be logical, practical, and work driven, not "impractical dreamers". The trouble with this type of thinking is that it keeps us from expanding our mind and therefore our experiences. If we limit ourselves to viewing our identity as strictly an individual separate from everything else in existence, we will remain separate and will feel unfulfilled. If we open our mind to a more expanded view of ourselves, we will give ourselves an opportunity to feel complete and whole. We are not just our ego, the part of ourselves that usually controls our life and our identity. The largest part of us, the most powerful and, ultimately, familiar part of us, is beyond our control. The idea that we don't control all of ourselves sets off an alarm to L-mode. Since we are so accustomed to using L-mode, we have a built in determination to stay in control, especially of something as personal and important to us as our identity. Our true nature comes from our source. This is the universally guided and organized energy of love. We are not in charge of this energy, but we can work with it as it guides us. We can allow ourselves or choose to feel this energy or not, but we did not create this energy. In order to discover or stay in touch with our true selves, we have to let go of our need to totally control our identity. We have to reshape the identity we've created to include an identity that trusts and surrenders to love. This is not only scary to L-mode, but it goes against its very nature. L-mode wants to be in charge rather than let our true self, the universal energy of love, be in charge. Resisting the idea that we are more than "take charge" entities requires consistent coaching and encouragement. It also requires remembering that you can't release L-mode's control over you unless you believe that L-mode exists and holds power over your thinking and perceptions of reality most of the time. L-mode is very powerful and very real, and it will stay in control of your thinking until you learn to expand your way of viewing.

Once you realize how controlling L-mode can be, you begin to see how it makes sense that we can trust love and know our true selves for a day or two and then change to feeling fear and aloneness. I'm not saying that L-mode is the enemy to love and spirit or that it is the only thing holding us back from trusting love and knowing our true selves more frequently and deeply, but I am saying that it plays a very large part in holding us back. What is required to maintain an inspired feeling of trust towards and a connection to love? Trusting love requires that we suspend disbelief and go with our instincts that urge us to keep moving in the direction of love. You have to be still in order to pick up the subtle messages of love, and you have to expect that you won't be disappointed. For all of our lives, we have been encouraged to stay in control and to remain guarded. If we follow these set patterns, we are letting go of an opportunity like no other. Letting go, in order to trust something subtle and unknown, is so opposite to what we've trained ourselves to do and what L-mode does best. If we trust that we do have a true self and are willing to let go of controlling everything, we will catch glimpses of an identity that far exceeds what we can now imagine.

Chances are, most of us have only a vague notion of spirit. Many people don't discuss or try to define their spirit in every-day life. What if you knew for certain that your true self, your spirit or universal love-based self, is very alive and knowable? Open your mind to this broader way of seeing by imagining that you can feel a core identity of love within you. Imagine that this core is so familiar that you feel like it was always there. Imagine that you have so much confidence and certainty about your life and yourself that you have no doubts, no regrets, no guilt, or pain, or fear. Imagine feeling so inspired that you easily form new ways of viewing and solving old problems. Imagine feeling completely heard, understood, and loved, so much so that you don't have to question or learn to trust the love. The love is just part of you. It is the foundation of your identity. When we can unite our ego identity or individual self with the source of love, we become capable of being the person I just described. This is our true self. Our true self carries all of our unique qualities and life experiences with it, but it unites us with the power and qualities of universal love. Love, our spirit, the universal source of energy, the essence of life, you can call it what you like, the point to be made is that we become empowered by it when we unite with it. When you realize that your identity is meant to be individual and universal, you begin to create your true self.

Our true self, the one that includes our individual identity and our universal identity, is the self we need to strive to be. If we understand that this is what we are meant to do, we can always keep moving in this direction. As we move along this path, we uncover obstacles and strengths that teach us where to step next. It is always a challenge to walk on a path when you don't know ahead of time exactly how you will get where you want to go, but this is how life is. We don't know what's around the corner most of the time. We can easily become discouraged if we worry too much about our unanswered questions or life's uncertainty.

Uncertainty is such a big part of life. It can create such fear and confusion in us. How often do we find ourselves wondering why something happened or what we should do? Almost every day we are faced with challenges that force us to deal with something that seems confusing or beyond our control. It is so easy to get distracted by all of these things. When something that is beyond your control occurs in your life, how do you respond? Of course this depends on the nature of what has occurred, but, in general, how do you respond to something that comes up out of the blue? How do you react when things don't go the way that you expected or desired? These are very important questions to ask ourselves on a regular basis because staying connected to our true self requires trusting uncertainty. We have to trust that our universal self will always be leading us, even when our ego or individual self can't figure out the plan. Most of the time, L-mode is in charge of how we perceive life, and L-mode hates surprises. If we ask ourselves how we respond to uncertainty, most of us would probably say that we don't like uncertainty. L-mode does not like disorder or unanswered questions. If something occurs that throws off our orderly, logical expectations and plans, L-mode panics. It wants things back the way we had intended them to be. L-mode's reaction to not having control is to force control on the situation. Have you ever noticed yourself trying to change something that just was never meant to be changed? For example, you may have expected to go to see a certain person or to attend a certain function and had organized your day around this event. When, for reasons beyond your control, the plan had to be cancelled, you tried to force things to change. Maybe you spent a lot of energy asking why things went the way they did, and maybe you got very frustrated or even angry because of being so disappointed or let down. When surprises occur or plans don't work the way we expected, our first response should be to ask if the unexpected situation was caused by something beyond our control. If we really did not cause the change, then we have to accept that it is quite possible that the change is meant to be. When we make our plans or go through each day, so often we end up being thrown off or confused by uncertainty or unexpected occurrences. Instead of trying to control what we can't control, turn off this L-mode way of viewing the situation and try to see it as an opportunity to learn something more about how you can trust the universe. Try to identify more with your universal self by trusting it. If you use R-mode and expand your view rather than stick to an L-mode controlling attitude, you can decrease your level of fear, frustration, and confusion. Uncertainty is part of life. If we let it make us feel fearful and frustrated, we are closing ourselves off from seeing it as an opportunity to increase our connection to our universal identity. Our universal identity has to be respected, and when we allow our fears and controlling L-mode ways to exist too frequently or intensely in our thoughts, we are limiting our connection to our true self. Uncertainty can be very frightening, but this is only because of having an L-mode response. R-mode will accept the uncertain and view it for what it is - something beyond our control.

This is such an important lesson to learn because we are so convinced that being in charge and having control is the most powerful place to exist. The truth is that staying connected to our universal identity gives us access to unlimited power. Trying to stay in charge of everything is the ego or individual self being separate from the universal self. L-mode convinces us that we are in a concrete reality, but we are also part of the universal reality. There is a larger system that extends beyond what occurs in our L-mode thoughts and our daily lives. The larger system extends beyond the concrete and organizes everything that exists. The universe is organized and operating at all times. It is alive within and outside of our personal lives, and it unites everything. Through energy, the universe vibrates and communicates on different levels and in different forms, and this energy always exists everywhere. We are connected to it. Even our overly controlling L-mode thoughts are part of the universal system. Universal energy exists in the expected and unexpected occurrences of our lives. It exists in the lives of our families and peers. It exists at every moment of every lifetime and in every section of every area of existence. Universal energy runs through and governs all that is. If we tune into the energy of the universe by accepting it as the foundation of our identity, we resonate with it in a more harmonious manner. We resist our connection to universal energy by feeling like separate or isolated individuals and by thinking that we are the only force guiding our lives. The force of the universe does guide our lives, and it points things out to us or gives us an awareness of or insights about how to resonate with life and love more easily. We are not supposed to believe that we need to be in complete charge of our lives. We are held responsible for our thoughts and actions, but we must give up our desire to control things so that we can allow ourselves to trust and be guided by the energy of the universe. The force of the universe has a plan. It is organized and is always functioning. Its plan is as alive as we are, and it should be recognized as a living thing rather than an abstract concept. If we train ourselves to experience the presence of the universe within us as a living, vibrating, life enhancing, organized system, L-mode will be forced to accept this energy as being real.

Uniting the plan of the universe with our own plans for ourselves does not have to be a huge challenge. Just give L-mode a rest. This lets you accept that even though you can't always see or touch the force of the universe, it does exist. Trying to accept the abstract is difficult if you forget that R-mode works with different rules than L-mode. R-mode imagination is key. If you imagine peace and love, R-mode says this experience makes peace and love real. If you imagine that the uncertainty in your life makes sense in a larger system than your own, R-mode allows you to experience and trust this expanded view. If you use R-mode to imagine love and to help you expand your thinking and your experiences of love, you will KNOW that no matter what happens, you can always trust that the peace will be there and that a feeling of connection to the universe can always be made. L-mode gets stuck or locked into the argument of whether or not the larger plan exists or is real. It loves to make a point and to have us work at something until we can disprove or prove it based on logic. How can we expect to KNOW the experience of suspending disbelief and trusting what is not concrete unless we nurture the qualities of R-mode perception? The shift from L-mode to R-mode perception must occur when we are faced with uncertainty. The logic of L-mode keeps us stuck in the frustration and confusion of uncertainty. R-mode is able to give us an opportunity to feel the subtle and accept the abstract. It gives us the opportunity to KNOW love and to develop our universal identity.

The universe is organized. It exists within us, and it exists within all of life. The organized energy that makes up the universe changes form and can be intensified or dulled depending on the intention of the observer. In other words, the energy of the universe, or love, is always there, but it becomes more obvious and increases in intensity for the observer when the observer chooses to see and trust the energy. What we choose to see and believe is what we will see and believe. If we feel that we are the recipient of an unfortunate occurrence that occurred because of something beyond our control, we can feel love and see opportunity or feel confusion and frustration, depending on what we choose to see. Ultimately, the freedom to choose how we perceive our reality is our greatest gift. Free will is a gift of being free to see and choose love. No matter what we have done, or how badly we feel, we can always choose to see love.

The universe created us and brought us to live in this world. It is responsible for our creation. When we remember this, we want to surrender to love, and we trust that the universe will guide and protect us. The universe already has given us so many things that are beyond our control like where we were born, the time or year in which we were born, the neighbors and school-mates we were given as a young child, the natural aptitudes and character traits we possess, the appearance of our physical form, our gender, our family, etc.. There are so many givens in life. We have been living under the direction of a larger system since we were born. When you look at it this way, it is much easier to give up some control and to remember to trust that the universe has a plan.

We have to remind ourselves that the unknown, uncertainty, and chance are not for L-mode analysis. Instead, we should be trying to experience these things with acceptance and an increased awareness of the existence of a universal plan. This does not mean that we have no choices in life and that all is pre-determined. We are meant to have our individual, choice mak-ing self unite with the universally guided part of our self. We don't have to lose our unique identity or surrender ourselves out of existence. We are meant to be a balance of individual and universal. This is what creates our true self.

We can know for certain that having an integrated universal and individual self brings the strengths of the universe to daily life. Not only do we calm our fears when we feel as though our identity is fundamentally a universal connection, but we increase our capacity to be certain of universal power, to think clearly, and to see opportunities rather than obstacles. The uni-versal part of us accepts all that exists. What happens, occurs for a reason. This helps take the pressure off us trying to constantly work at fixing everything. Things can be in a mess, but when you remember your universal nature, you will feel empowered and confident.

Once we are aware of how to tap into our universal identity, we receive strengths we normally would not possess. When you remember that you are not just your personality, the parent, the spouse, the employer, the employee, and the member of a community and society, etc. and include the feeling of belonging to a universal plan, you are given insights and guidance to aid you in your life. The universe is organized by intelligence, wisdom, truth, order, clarity and all the qualities you would associate with a highly enlightened person. The universe communicates with and guides us by using or giving us these same qualities. When you receive an insight or have a very clear idea, the universe is communicating with you. At these times, you are strengthening your connection to your true self. If you are given a wonderful feeling of awe and appreciation because of seeing something beautiful in nature or in another person, the universe is communicating with you and drawing your identity back towards its fundamental nature. Every time you feel appreciation and love, you are connecting to your true self. These experiences should be sought after and respected because they unite us with the universe. If you watch a beautiful movie, or read an eloquent passage in a book, or absorb a new concept that makes you sigh with peace and comfort, remember that you are intensifying your relationship with your true self. If you watch graceful and artistic dancing or incredible athletic performances and feel united with the performer and the performance through appreciation and respect, you are uniting with the energy that unites all that exists. Artistic and athletic performances of beauty capture our attention so passionately because they are expressions of universal truths. We are drawn to them because they cause us to remember or resonate with our fundamental nature. Our true self is connected to love in all its expressions, so experiencing love through beauty in any form causes our soul to become more familiar.

The voice of the universe is love. When we learn to search for it, we can see that it speaks in many forms. One form is what some people refer to as their instincts or inner voice. When we want to connect to our inner voice, the quality we search for is a sense of rightness or a knowing or certainty that love is at the root of the issue or thought we are questioning. If we want to know what to do at any given moment, we have a guidance center that we can consult at any time. It is easy to access once you know what you are looking for. Learning to pay attention to this gut level response is an important part of the process of growing closer to our true selves. If we sit still and ask ourselves the question we need answered, we can learn to recognize the subtle but very clear answers that come from our instincts in the form of certainty and knowing. We can know for sure if something is right or wrong for us at a particular moment in our lives if we sit still and listen. If we relax our L-mode thinking and ask the question, we will get a response of great certainty. If something feels right for us, we will resonate with it or feel peaceful about it. If something feels wrong, we will sense turmoil or discomfort on an emotional and even on a physical level.

Our inner voice is our instincts telling us what to do. It serves to protect us, and it draws us closer to our universal self. The universe has messages for us, and when we use R-mode to slow down, to be aware of the moment, and to become absorbed in and fascinated by the subtle, we can sense the messages from our inner voice. The voice is not an actual sound. It is an intuitive or instinctive knowing that what we have just sensed or experienced feels right or wrong. Connection to this part of ourselves is something we can increase so that we can approach each day with the constant readiness to being alerted by our instincts. By giving cues of emotion and insight, our instincts help us connect the details of our life with the plan of the universe. When we learn to trust our instincts, we feel the guidance of the universe in our lives. This helps us to be less fearful of uncertainty and to remain fixed on the idea that we are not alone. We exist as individuals with unique experiences and qualities and with the freedom to choose. We also exist as part of the universe. The larger system carries us within itself. We are part of the larger system of life, and we are meant to stay connected to and be guided by this system.

Love and beauty surround us at all times. They are always available to be noticed and absorbed. The more intensely we search for love, the more love we will find. Love is the unifying force of the universe. It gives us a way of staying connected to everything in existence and a way to not be afraid of what seems unfair or what is unknowable. Uncertainty, pain, loneliness, and fear are part of life. We are able and meant to rise above these things. When we remember to search for love and think of it as part of our identity, and choose to trust the universe rather than control our lives, we discover our entire self. Our entire self is individual and universal.

CHAPTER 9

Letting Go

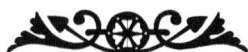

A ccepting and trusting our universal self takes time and patience. Since we are operating with L-mode perception most of the time, trusting and accepting the subtle is usually quite difficult. How can we get around our tendency to stay in control at all times? How can we train ourselves to let go? We do this with the help of R-mode and with a greater understanding of the energy of love.

Letting go is the most challenging aspect of maintaining a connection to our universal identity. Letting go requires that we trust or act on faith. Everyone knows how difficult it is to remember faith let alone have faith when we are in the middle of a crisis. Faith requires that we suspend our fears and disbelief in order to leave room for love and peace. A faith filled heart is a love filled heart. Fear and disbelief represent our controlling side. The L-mode part of us hates to let go and has a very powerful voice in our mind. Logic and control create a controlling type of reaction to crisis and even every day life. The main point to remember is that we have different modes of perceiving reality or life. We can approach things with L-mode or R-mode tendencies. Each way produces very different results, and we are able to be in charge of choosing our mode of perception. Since L-mode is usually dominant, we can say with almost complete certainty that we have to train ourselves to choose R-mode more often. We are already very adept at being logical and believing the concrete, empirical evidence we see in front of us. We are already very good at being reasonable and taking charge of situations through analysis and orderly planning. We are not; however, good at letting go in order to let something abstract solve our problems. R-mode gives great value to the abstract, subtle reality, and R-mode is our ally when it comes to training ourselves to remain faith filled. R-mode will assist us when we try to suspend our disbelief and fears and when we try to create room for love.

Faith requires letting go in order to allow love and the plan of the universe do its job. Love must enter chaos in order to rebuild it into order. If we don't let go, how will there be room for love to enter the situation? We can be looking at a situation outside of ourselves, within our mind, or one that is a combination of both of these things, but the same rule always applies. How can we expect order to be created if we don't make room for love to enter? The universe has the power to incorporate love and order into any situation, but our union with love is how we must assist the universe. If we want everything to happen as the universe intended, or if we want to have our lives unite with a universal plan, we need to unite with love and release L-mode control. Letting go is allowing ourselves to trust love. It can occur in various ways, but most often letting go requires that we drop our controlling L-mode attitude and shift to a calm, peaceful R-mode approach.

Letting go frees up energy and lets if flow. This energy can be thought of as physical energy, emotional energy, and the intellectual energy of thought. It can be looked at as the under-lying source of all that exists. Everything that exists is inter-acting and communicating on very subtle energy levels. We are bound with everything that exists through this subtle energy. This energy, in its most basic or fundamental form, exists always and everywhere. It changes its form and intensity, but it is at the core of our thoughts, our emotions, and our physical reality. Love is a way to describe this energy, but keep in mind that this is a big concept. We don't have many words to describe the various forms of this energy, so "love" is being used here to describe something more complex than our everyday under-standing of love.

The most common way of identifying love is to describe it as an emotion of the heart that unites us with what we appreci-ate. When we respect and appreciate something, we feel drawn towards it and want to unite with it. Because of these desires and responses, we can experience intense emotional feelings and physical sensations. When we feel a platonic or mate based love for someone, it can be said that this person or our love for them opens up our heart or warms our heart. Falling in love can make our heart "skip a beat" or cause our heart to pound. There are so many references to love that include a reference to physical sensations, especially ones that are centered around the heart. We can lose our breath and feel very emotionally affected by our physical reactions to love. All of these reactions, both emotional and physical, can be viewed with L-mode logic or they can be seen through a more open-minded view with the help of R-mode perception. If we look at the responses we have to love as the energy of love passing through our emo-tions and physical body, love can be understood with more of an expanded view. Imagine the feelings and physical sensations of love, and think of them as energy traveling through you. This energy increases if you allow the love to flow freely. This is what I mean by "letting go" - thinking of love as energy and letting it flow without resistance. When we let ourselves trust the love, and it flows with greater intensity, and we feel the effects of this increased intensity through our thoughts and emotions and through various physical sensations, we are surrendering or letting go to love. If we don't let go because we can't or won't trust the love, we create energy blocks, and we cut ourselves off from the powerful effects of love. Love is meant to be energy in motion. It is meant to flow through our bodies, emotions, and minds. It is able to intensify itself and therefore its affect on us when we let go and allow it to flow freely.

Remember the examples I just gave of reactions to falling in love? Well, imagine the opposite to these reactions. Imagine being afraid to love. What would your thoughts, your emotions, and your body feel like if you did not trust love or the person you wanted to love? Your body, especially your heart, would feel fixed or closed. At times in my life, as I'm sure is the case with most people, I have felt like there was a wall around my heart. The fear we can feel towards letting go to love can come from many different past experiences. The results of not letting go to love are usually the same. It causes physical reactions in our body, reactions in our thoughts, and emotional reactions. We can think fearful thoughts, or we can feel fear and pain, and our heart can become cold or blocked or closed. We hear the term "cold hearted" associated with someone behaving in a loveless manner, but all of us are able to be closed and open hearted or warm and cold hearted. These are ways of describing a physical sensation and an emotional response. Our heart area has the power to expand in some sense. We can open our heart and let love flow through, or we can close our heart and resist the flow of love. Most of us are able to feel open and loving in many areas of our lives, and we open and close our heart, to different degrees, depending on the mood we are in or the situation we are facing. What is missing from common knowledge about love is a discussion of how to open our heart. If you focus on opening your heart to allow love to flow through it, you are learning to "let go". If you use R-mode to imagine your heart as a focus point for love, and treat love as an energy that needs to flow, you increase your power to allow love to flow through you. When we allow the feeling of love to be sensed by us as an energy flowing through our heart, we not only increase the physical and emotional intensity of experiencing love, but we begin to think loving thoughts. By unblocking the energy of love in our heart, we open the door to all the strengths of love. Love brings clarity of mind, confidence, certainty, etc. If we want to acquire more of the strengths of love, we can remember that love is an energy that must flow, and we stop the flow and start the flow through our understanding of letting go.

Love, when it is free to flow through the heart, affects us physically in various ways. When our heart is filled and flowing with love, we feel relaxed. We may find ourselves sighing, and we may feel like expanding our chest or breathing deeper and standing taller. When we allow love to let us feel filled or expanded physically in our body or chest area, we can encourage this expansion by using R-mode. Imagine, after you open your heart or expand it with love, that you are "letting go" in your entire body and are first expanding the love or letting it flow within your lungs. Letting energy, calm and peaceful, subtle energy flow through your chest and neck area will increase your experience of love. It may sound odd to move from describing love of the heart, "falling in love type love", to love of the lungs, but keep an open mind. Use R-mode rather than L-mode logic. When you think of or sense love as a flowing energy, you are giving yourself an opportunity to direct the peaceful energy through your body. The lungs want to expand when you feel love, so allow them to expand. Let go and let the energy flow. The emotional effect you experience from letting the energy of love flow to the rest of the body is not exactly the same as what you feel from love in your heart area, but it is similar. Letting the love you feel in your heart expand and relax your heart brings intense emotional feelings of joy and peace. When you let this energy flow through your chest, neck, spine, head, and down to your abdomen, etc., these emotions are not as present, but your body does relax, and you do feel peaceful. By letting the energy of love flow through your body, you are allowing yourself to become more closely aware of how the energy of the universe is part of your body. We are connected to the universe through our heart and mind but also through our body.

When your body is tense, it causes energy, subtle universal healing energy, to be unable to flow through those areas. The goal in healing ourselves or in living is to live to our greatest physical, emotional, mental, and spiritual potential. Our physical body is part of the universe. All that exists is, at its core, made of universal energy, so our body will respond to love. Our body will relax and work with greater health and efficiency if we connect to it through its fundamental nature of loving energy. We don't have to look at our body as being separate from universal love. Our body is made of the energy of the universe. When I feel love, universal awe inspired love, my body reacts. I become aware of my heart, I feel it pulsating, I feel heat in my chest area, etc.. Our bodies respond to love or the unifying energy of the universe because they are made of this energy at their core level.

Tension in our body is causing blocks that won't allow universal energy to flow through us. Our bodies work best when we are able to get rid of our tension blocks. By concentrating on different areas of tension and trying to transport the loving energy you feel in your heart to these areas of tension, you unblock them and clear a path for universal energy to flow. Letting go in our body increases our connection to and awareness of loving energy.

This same idea can be applied to our thinking. If you get stuck in fearful thoughts that repeat themselves over and over in your mind, you are creating a block. Negative thinking creates a block in the sense that it keeps us from being open to loving thoughts. Love needs to flow freely. When it comes across a block, it can't heal or influence the blocked area without us choosing to let go in this area. Working through these points of tension requires that we let go of them. We replace the negative thoughts with loving thoughts.

Love needs a path to flow through. When our bodies, emotions, or thoughts create a block, we should focus on these areas and bring love to them. Releasing, or letting go physically, emotionally, and mentally teaches us to trust the universe. It increases our faith in love. It helps us to realize that the subtle realty of love can have a very concrete and real impact on our lives.

Life is always offering us opportunities to expand our thinking and to create a new, more fulfilling reality for ourselves.

Letting go of old ways of viewing things and old habits that don't encourage us to heal and grow is so essential in life. Letting go of control and opening up to trust is the way of spiritual evolution, and it can be done on many levels.

A big part of letting go is realizing how easy it is to stay stuck in patterns of thinking. How many times do we find ourselves concerned with things that we can't control? If something occurred in our past, whether it is because of us or because of something someone else did, we have to learn to let it go. It's difficult to change habitual thought patterns and reactions, but it is necessary. If we stay angry or upset at ourselves or others for past actions, universal energy is not being allowed to flow through the thought/situation. This does not promote healing and growth. A very common example of this is holding on to excessive guilt. Guilt becomes a negative influence over us when we feel it too often or too extremely. Of course we should pay attention to our emotions of guilt and remorse to a certain degree. They are there to teach us how and when we need to change our behavior, but these emotions can easily become too extreme. Since we are driven by a desire to accomplish things, and L-mode loves accomplishments, any deviation from our set goals can cause us to be self-critical. Guilt is a strong emotion, and when you couple that with our L-mode tendency to expect perfection, we can end up being way too self-critical. L-mode locks on to judgment very easily. Our logical side is built to judge and criticize, so when we are judging ourselves, we have to be very aware of how easy it is to get stuck in this L-mode task. We are more than our L-mode view of ourselves. We are able to let go of a negative, self-critical view of our thoughts and actions if we shift to R-mode. R-mode sees the bigger picture.

It allows us to expand our views. Guilt becomes unhealthy if we stay stuck in L-mode self-criticism, and we can release excessive guilt by expanding our view of ourselves.

We are given a guidance center to help us sense when something is right or wrong for us. Our instincts or inner voice is our messenger from the spirit realm. If we are able to pay attention to and follow its guidance, we become aware of what is right and wrong for our spiritual growth. Guilt is meant to be a healthy emotion that sets in when we have not followed our instincts. Our inner voice speaks to us through guilt when we have not followed what is best for our spiritual evolution. So, when we feel guilty, should we see it as simply a sign to examine our choices, or should we use L-mode to increase our feelings of guilt. Should we thank our inner voice for getting our attention and examine our situation with the intention of making the necessary changes and releasing our guilt, or should we get angry at ourselves and remain stuck in guilty feelings. It is obvious that staying stuck in the negative emotions of excessive guilt is not going to help us to grow.

Our tendency is to think that if we make mistakes, we are failing. This is a logical way of viewing things. Why can't we see that we are works in progress? If we open up our mind to include the idea that we are here to learn, we will accept our imperfections. L-mode wants perfection and constant order, but life and people are not perfect. We are constantly learning and growing. That is just the way of life. We are created to become aware of our spiritual essence, and when we forget our essence, we make mistakes. They cannot be looked at as right and wrong in an L-mode sense of perfection. Mistakes are right and wrong in relationship to our growth. A mistake is a lesson.

It exists to remind us of our spiritual essence. It is not an indication that we are unworthy of being spiritual creatures. If you
accept that you and your life are not perfect and that that is the
way it is meant to be, you will find it easier to let go of excessive self-criticism. Letting go of excessive guilt and self-criticism
allows you to keep moving forward. When we get stuck because
we forget that we are not supposed to be or are not expected to
be perfect, our R-mode can help us out. Use an open-minded,
"in the moment" approach to replace judgment and to place
loving thoughts in your mind. R-mode gives us the accepting,
open-minded attitude we need when we forget that it's o.k. to
be imperfect. Let the love you are capable of feeling flow to your
opinion of yourself. Let go of your self-criticism by allowing
love to enter.

Forgiving ourselves for our mistakes is an extremely freeing
process. When we forgive ourselves, we open up our heart to
loving ourselves. This reminds us that we are spiritual creatures.
We know or become familiar with or identify with our spiritual
self much more intensely when we concentrate on loving ourselves. It is relatively easy to say or to understand intellectually
that we are spiritual creatures, but we really can't know our
spiritual nature until we experience or feel love for ourselves.
Learning to love ourselves is a process that involves recognizing
that we are not meant to be perfect, recognizing that mistakes
are necessary in order to change and grow, and realizing that
self-forgiveness is the key to feeling love for ourselves. When we
open our heart and forgive ourselves and accept ourselves just as
we are, we allow love to enter and flow through us. This encourages us to get rid of the ideas that we have formed about our
identity being defined based on harsh judgment of ourselves.

Our true identity is grounded in spiritual awareness. Our spirit is rooted in the energy of the universe. We are not our mistakes, our imperfections, our wrong actions and short comings. We are meant to be more than these things. We are meant to feel love and to relate to love as the main part of our identity.

The same idea applies to forgiving and accepting others. We have to realize that everyone's essential nature is spiritual. If we see everyone as a vibrating center of spiritual energy, this becomes their identity. If we focus on the hurts they've caused us or the flaws in their character, these negative qualities will become what we see as their identity. Remembering that the same universe that created us created everyone else is very helpful. The universe is bound together through love and acceptance. All that is created can vibrate in harmony with the universe. When we accept the things we encounter on the basis of their spiritual essence, we are encouraging ourselves and these things to vibrate more harmoniously with the universal energy of love. When we criticize or stay angry at someone, we are causing disharmony for ourselves and others. Acceptance does not mean that you ignore the negative behavior of the other person, it just means that you forgive them and that you refuse to define them by that behavior. By letting go of anger and criticism towards others, you open up an area for love to enter. If we don't give love towards others room to exist, we will not be in touch with the essential or purest nature of each person we encounter. When we focus on love, and then direct this towards others, we see love in them. We realize that they are essentially the same as us, and this act creates a bond or flow of energy.

Forgiveness is achieved by choosing love. We can forgive ourselves and others when we let go of our guilt and anger, etc.

by allowing love to enter our mind and heart. We do this by letting R-mode expand the situation. This, in turn, forces L-mode criticism and judgment to stop. R-mode allows us to see and feel love in the moment and to refrain from being overly judgmental. If you train yourself to use R-mode to see the beauty in nature or any other thing you enjoy, you can train yourself to use R-mode to see the beauty in others.

Accepting and trusting love takes courage and practice. When we choose to accept and trust love, to feel love in our heart, and to let this energy flow, we are given the power of love. Our own behavior, the behavior of others, the unexpected events of our lives, uncertainty, etc., give us opportunities to open up to love.

We can train ourselves to release control and let go by recognizing that love is always where we must turn. If our heart feels closed, we need to let go and physically feel love in our heart. If our body is tight and reacting to stress and fear, we need to send loving energy through our body. If our L-mode thoughts are controlling and/or overly critical, we need to let those thoughts go, by shifting to R-mode perception. Becoming more open-minded stops L-mode judgment and control. We need to create room for loving thoughts to enter. Let go and let love enter. We can use R-mode and an ever increasing understanding of the energy of love to help us to let go and go with the flow of love. Our focus should always be love.

CHAPTER 10

Changing Focus

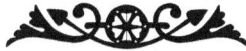

The most helpful lesson I've learned in my life time is that L-mode dominates too many of our thoughts and perceptions. Knowing this and learning how to change my focus to more of an R-mode approach to life has given me a closer connection to my spirit. My aim in writing this book has been to share what I have learned. I hope that you can and will continue to relate to some of my experiences and interpretations of spiritual growth.

We use L-mode to guide our thoughts and actions most of the time, but L-mode runs on logical thinking. The biggest drawback to using logical thought too frequently is that it prevents us from accepting what we can't prove logically. How important is it to learn to trust what you can't always see? Isn't that the essence of maintaining faith in love? L-mode does not want to harm us, but it does harm us when it causes us to forget that too much logic keeps us removed from faith. Too much logic causes us to forget that what we can't see clearly and describe in logical terms has to have merit. Changing focus from L-mode to R-mode helps us to maintain our faith. Logic says that faith has to be reserved for explainable experiences.

R-mode lets us take the leap. It gives us room or a mind-set that is willing to suspend judgment and logic because that feels like the right thing to do. Changing focus from L-mode to R-mode is one of the most powerful things we can do to increase our faith in universal love. What we focus on, and how we interpret situations, depends directly on what mode of perception we are using. When it comes to things as important as our questions of sensing and trusting the love of the universe, or trying to maintain faith, logical thoughts will hold us back. Logic is not what we should use as our system of proof that love always exists. It's a difficult thing to accept, but logic, and other L-mode ways of thinking and perceiving, can actually decrease our faith. During the times when we need to be strong and to remember faith, we have to observe how we are focusing our mind. Are we using L-mode or R-mode to interpret our situation? If we know that the two modes exist, if we try to develop R-mode, and if we try to decrease our overuse of L-mode, we have given ourselves very powerful tools to assist us in our spiritual growth.

Surrendering to a life that feels guided by universal love, rather than trying to control life, is another change in focus that we can practice. We can arrive in a position where we are not focused on the struggle of life but instead are focused on the guidance life gives. Surrendering is an attitude. It comes about when you realize that you are going to be ok if you let go of control and hold on to love. L-mode wants to control, and R-mode wants to experience and feel. It trusts what it feels, so if you want to learn to trust and surrender to love, you have to let yourself feel love. We may, on some level, understand that love is there to help us, but L-mode discourages us from always remembering this because it wants to control rather than surrender. L-mode can't see the logic in letting go of controlling everything in our life. Logically, it does not make sense to step back and wait for guidance. L-mode wants us to do things quickly and efficiently. It believes we are wasting time and are going to lose if we are not always on top of everything. It thinks it has to control life and not let go. The only way around this is to shift to R-mode. Don't wait for L-mode to believe in and trust the universe. Change your focus to feelings of love and a sense of guidance and try to gradually let go of controlling thoughts. Changing focus from feeling driven by control to focusing on expecting guidance, following intuition, and feeling and trusting love requires less L-mode and more R-mode. As I just said, R-mode trusts what it feels, so if you want to learn to trust and surrender to love, you have to let yourself feel love. Use R-mode. Relax, imagine, and then feel love. When we change our focus to feelings and thoughts of love and the beauty of the moment, we begin learning how to trust and surrender to love. Once we begin to trust love, we will find it much easier to let our lives be guided by the universe.

Timing is also a concept we should consider in the context of changing focus. Because of our dominant L-mode, we like to hurry and be organized and efficient with our thoughts and lives. Even if these actions cause us to feel tired and stuck in unhealthy patterns, L-mode keeps pushing us to hurry and get things done. This is a huge benefit, and a necessity one, if it is done in moderation, but if we are so driven by time that we expect everything to happen quickly and/or on our schedule, we can't be feeling connected to or accepting of the timing of the universe. The universe has a plan. It is organized and efficient, but the timing of the universe is not necessarily our timing. We tend to move too quickly and expect things to happen quickly. The universe lets things happen when it is time for them to happen. Often, we expect ourselves to accomplish things and to meet goals we have set for ourselves without deep reflection on whether or not we are truly ready to have these things occur. The universe lets things occur to us when we are ready for them to occur. If we change our focus from expecting our timing to be the best timing, to letting the universe give us what we need when it feels we are ready, we will save ourselves a lot of anguish. Universal time is more abstract than L-mode wants it to be. L-mode loves to know present and future details down to the exact hour and minute and/or day and month. It loves being aware of the exact time. This is a natural and healthy quality, to a degree. We need to have schedules and to synchronize our lives in order to stay in touch with others and our responsibilities, etc., but if we stay too focused on this type of rigid, precise timing, we can forget to see the big picture. The universe holds the big picture. Universal time moves according to readiness. There is a time for everything, according to the universe, and it will not be governed by watches and dates. Universal time is more spread out and abstract. The passage of days and years is not the main issue with the universal system. This L-mode concern with the passage of time is how we usually relate to time. The universal system runs with more of an R-mode approach. Time passage is not really noticed. The universal system concerns itself with the transformation and movement of spiritual energy. When we are feeling and experiencing universal love, we can relate to not being concerned with the passage of time. During any intense R-mode moment, time is forgotten. R-mode places us "in the moment" and draws our attention to experiencing all of the subtle beauty of that moment. That experience can be referred to as "being". The universe is in a constant state of "being". That is why it is not entering, judging, or categorizing our lives based on L-mode time related values. It is organized, but it works with and through our lives while "being". The plan of the universe unfolds in accordance with the readiness of everyone and everything involved. If we are spiritually aware of ourselves, we can more easily sense when we are ready for things to occur. Maybe we feel ready but other people or situations are not. We have to accept this as part of the universal plan. If we try to stay focused on our spiritual self, our timing desires will eventually synchronize more closely with universal timing. In other words, we won't question universal timing. We will adopt the attitude that everything happens for a reason.

When things don't happen at the time we believe they should happen, we can step back and ask ourselves if we are spiritually prepared for the moment to occur. I'm sure everyone can recall several or maybe many things that happened later in their life than they had hoped. When we look back at them, it is often easy to see that those things occurred at exactly the right moment to assist us in learning an important spiritual lesson. It is so easy to become impatient with life when things don't go the way we think they should go, but we have the choice to change focus to universal time. "Being in the moment" really helps us to move with and accept universal timing.

The universe is in a state of "being", and the more we step into that "being" state, the more attached we become to the universe. The "being" state is the state of being in love. When we are "being", we feel love. The love is not a thought, it is a physical feeling in our heart. Many people are confused about how to "be" in love. They don't realize that love is alive, it's an action, it moves you, and it feels real. Just as you can be near your mate all day but not be drawn to them, you can believe in the love of the universe and yet not be drawn to it. The reverse situation, where you can have a day with your mate where you do feel bonded to them, is one of "being" in love. You are drawn to them, you want to tell them you love them, and you are happy to be playful with them and to be near them. Many new couples feel this bliss. They are in love and can feel it as a very real feeling. It feels like a physical bond. So, the point I am making is that the state of "being" is as real as the state of "being in love" with your mate. If we want to evolve spiritually, we must make sure that we get the point that "being" or really feeling love is how we connect to and resonate with our spirit and the universe. We can read and discuss and think through many valuable concepts, but until we learn how to "be in love" we are missing a big piece of the puzzle.

The notion of "being" is the running theme of this book. I understand that I am not revealing something new. "Being" is a concept that is widely discussed. The position I bring to this discussion is that L-mode thinking is a major part of what prevents us from "being". R-mode is the "in the moment" state, and as I have said already, R-mode is not familiar enough to most people. L-mode is naturally aggressive and will overtake our attention. R-mode is naturally slow and gentle. "Being" requires more of an R-mode approach, so not knowing that R-mode exists or exactly what it is, and not knowing how to shift to R-mode can make "being" very difficult. L-mode thinking is where we spend much of our time. Hence the title of this book: "Changing Focus - From Left Brain Thinking to Right Brain "Being".

All of the chapters in this book were written to help the reader understand this main point. We are not really living and experiencing the splendor and power of spiritual evolution unless we know how and when to turn off our L-mode thinking and how to "be" in love. I revealed this main idea in pieces, and I tried to take care not to throw in too many abstract ideas all at once. What follows is a brief summary of each chapter. I have written them to try and help clarify the main points of each chapter and to show more directly why we need to change focus from L-mode thinking to R-mode "being".

Chapter 1: Love Is Our Purpose

Yes, we are here to discover love in as many different ways as we can. Love is our fundamental nature. It governs our spirit and all of life, and it is what unites us with the universe. Our ultimate purpose is to "be" in love, to enter, identify with, and exist in the feeling of love.

Chapter 2 Right Brain/Left Brain

They exist. Essentially, I wanted to introduce the brain modes right away because that is what this story is about. They exist, and most people don't have a clue that they do exist.

Chapter 3 Creativity

The process, not the product, of creativity is not understood or valued as it should be. We have to treat our journey through life as a creative process because that is what it means to "be". "Being" is a creative process. "Being" requires that we suspend judgment, that we give our lives time to develop, that we trust our instincts and learn to not control the process, that we search for and feel beauty and experience the use of imagination and the inspiration of an open, clear, insightful mind. Understanding the creative mind and the creative process helps us learn about how to stay in a state of "being".

Chapter 4 L-Mode Thinking
We think too much with L-mode. We are too logical, too analytical, too judgmental, and too control hungry to allow ourselves to live a "creative process" life. "Being" requires that we use less L-mode.

Chapter 5 The Subtle Reality of Existence
There is a subtle realm. It exists within our lives. When we enter this realm, we see beauty and purpose in all of existence. We enter this realm when we are "being".

Chapter 6 Negative Influences
Negative influences pull us away from "being".

Chapter 7 Loneliness and Being Alone
We have to face our fundamental loneliness because if we don't, we will find it very difficult to be alone. If we want to identify more closely with our spirit, we need to spend time alone.

Chapter 8 Our True Selves
When we contact our spiritual nature frequently enough, eventually, we begin to relate to it as the main part of our identity.

Chapter 9 Letting Go

Letting go requires releasing the physical, emotional, and mental blocks that prevent us from going with the flow of love. If our purpose is to love, to discover, relate to, and feel love to a point where we identify with it and realize that we are love, letting go of all the things that impede the flow of love is our order of business. Being in love, feeling love, relating to and identifying with love are achieved gradually through a gentle, creative process, but letting go and letting love flow can be done at any moment on a physical, emotional, and intellectual level.

Chapter 10 Changing Focus

I have given a reminder of and new slants on points I have already addressed, namely that we should change focus from L-mode to R-mode, from control to surrender, and from our timing to universal timing.

I am very grateful to have been given the opportunity to have this experience. The points I have written about have been life changers for me and continue to teach me different ways in which I can evolve spiritually. The main things I remind myself of are how important it is to stay focused on love, how necessary it is to keep love alive and real so that I am "being" in love, and how the process of creativity is a method I must respect and understand so that I can use it to help myself "be".

Too much L-mode pulls me away from "being", so changing my focus from L-mode to R-mode has become my guide.

www.ingramcontent.com/pod-product-compliance
Lightning Source LLC
Chambersburg PA
CBHW051735020426
42333CB00014B/1321